Immunochemistry in Clinical Laboratory Medicine

Immunochemistry in Clinical Laboratory Medicine

Edited by
A. Milford Ward
and
J. T. Whicher

Proceedings of a symposium
held at the University of Lancaster,
March, 1978

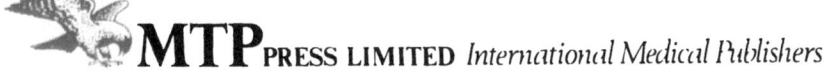

MTPPRESS LIMITED *International Medical Publishers*

Published by
MTP Press Limited
Falcon House
Cable Street
Lancaster, England

Copyright © 1979 MTP Press Limited

Softcover reprint of the hardcover 1st edition 1979

ISBN-13: 978-94-011-6593-8   e-ISBN-13: 978-94-011-6591-4

DOI: 10.1007/978-94-011-6591-4

Northgate, Blackburn, Lancs BB2 1AB

Contents

List of Contributors   ix

Preface   xi

SECTION ONE

Methods and Problems in Immunochemistry
Chairmen: Dr A. Milford Ward and Dr A. R. Bradwell

1   **Electrophoresis and immunoelectrophoresis**   3
Pamela G. Riches

2   **Radial immunodiffusion and rocket immunoelectrophoresis**   17
D. Kenny

3   **Automated immunoprecipitation and laser nephelometry**   23
P. A. E. White and R. Strong

4   **Antiserum requirements**   35
A. C. Munro

5   **Problems encountered in immunochemical technique methodology**   51
J. T. Whicher

6   **Specific protein measurement and standardization**   63
R. S. Wainwright, J. R. Doggart and D. W. Neill

7   **Quality control**   75
D. M. Browning

SECTION TWO

Specific Proteins in Laboratory Diagnosis
*Chairmen: Mr D. M. Browning, Dr R. S. H. Pumphrey,
Dr J. Kohn, Professor J. Hardwicke and Dr A. C. Munro*

8   **Structure and function of the immunoglobulins**   **85**
    R. S. H. Pumphrey

9   **Immunoglobulins in blood transfusion**   **99**
    P. D. J. Holt

10 **Monoclonal proteins**   **115**
    J. Kohn

11 **Iron binding proteins**   **127**
    A. Jacobs

12 **Albumin**   **135**
    Linda Smith

13 **The complement system**   **149**
    J. T. Whicher

14 **Alphafetoprotein in obstetrics**   **165**
    D. J. H. Brock

15 **Alphafetoprotein in oncology**   **177**
    J. Kohn

16 **α_1-Antitrypsin**   **183**
    A. Milford Ward

17 **Haptoglobin and orosomucoid in lung and breast
    tumours**   **197**
    A. R. Bradwell

SECTION THREE

Immunochemistry of Other Body Fluids
Chairman: Dr J. T. Whicher

18 Urinary proteins   **219**
    J. Hardwicke

19 Immunochemistry of CSF proteins   **229**
    E. J. Thompson

    Discussion   **237**

    Index   **243**

List of Contributors

Dr A. R. BRADWELL
Immunodiagnostics Research Laboratory, University of Birmingham

Dr D. J. H. BROCK
Department of Human Genetics, University of Edinburgh

Mr D. M. BROWNING
Wolfson Research Laboratory, Department of Clinical Chemistry, Queen Elizabeth Medical Centre, Birmingham

Mr J. R. DOGGART
Department of Biochemistry, Royal Victoria Hospital, Belfast

Professor J. HARDWICKE
Department of Immunology, University of Birmingham

Mr P. D. J. HOLT
Immunochemistry Laboratory, South West Regional Transfusion Centre, Bristol

Professor A. JACOBS
Department of Haematology, University Hospital of Wales, Cardiff

Mr D. KENNY
Department of Biochemistry, Our Lady's Hospital for Sick Children, Dublin

Dr J. KOHN
Supraregional Protein Reference Unit, Putney General Hospital, London

Dr A. C. MUNRO
Glasgow and West of Scotland Blood Transfusion Service, Law Hospital, Carluke, Lanarkshire

Mr D. W. NEILL
Department of Biochemistry, Royal Victoria Hospital, Belfast

Dr R. S. H. PUMPHREY
Department of Immunology, St Mary's Hospital, Manchester

Dr PAMELA G. RICHES
Supraregional Protein Reference Unit, Westminster Hospital Medical School, London

Dr LINDA SMITH
Department of Biochemistry, Hull Royal Infirmary, Hull

Mr R. STRONG
Supraregional Protein Reference Unit, Hallamshire Hospital, Sheffield

Dr E. J. THOMPSON
Department of Chemical Pathology, National Hospital for Nervous Diseases, Queen's Square, London

Dr A. MILFORD WARD
Supraregional Protein Reference Unit, Hallamshire Hospital, Sheffield

Mr R. S. WAINWRIGHT
Department of Biochemistry, Royal Victoria Hospital, Belfast

Dr J. T. WHICHER
Department of Chemical Pathology, Bristol Royal Infirmary, Bristol

Mr P. A. E. WHITE
Supraregional Protein Reference Unit, Hallamshire Hospital, Sheffield

Preface

The rapid growth of specific protein estimations in the clinical laboratory over the last 10 years has been due to advances both in methodology and in the understanding of the role of the various plasma proteins in health and disease. This expansion has been made possible by the development of both gel phase and fluid phase techniques for the estimation of proteins and the ready availability of antisera to individual plasma proteins. The specificity of the immunological reaction has allowed the more precise identification and estimation of individual plasma proteins than was possible with dye binding or other chemical techniques, but at the same time these methods have introduced other possible errors and pitfalls.

Advances in understanding of the structure and function of various plasma proteins has pointed the way to new clinical applications of plasma protein estimation in the diagnosis and monitoring of disease.

The Symposium, of which these are the proceedings, was planned to bring together a number of experts in the field to discuss the available methods and their clinical application.

The first part of the Symposium was devoted to methodology and dealt with techniques, reagent supply and control, and the various problems which might arise in the routine clinical laboratory. The second, and larger, part of the Symposium was devoted to a discussion of the clinical relevance of some of the more commonly estimated plasma proteins. The scope of the discussion was enlarged to include proteins in urine and cerebrospinal fluid. It was not the intention of the Symposium to discuss all the possible uses of immunochemistry in relation to clinical laboratory medicine but simply to highlight some of the advantages and disadvantages of immunochemical methods for the estimation of certain plasma proteins and to put these into a proper perspective in relation to modern clinical laboratory practice.

The contributors and editors are deeply grateful to the Hyland Division of Travenol Laboratories Limited who sponsored the Symposium and provided the administrative services needed to run it. The editors acknowledge the helpful collaboration of our publisher, and of Mrs. Judy Fagelston who transcribed the discussions.

SECTION ONE

Methods and Problems in Immunochemistry

Chairmen: Dr A. Milford Ward and Dr A. R. Bradwell

1

Electrophoresis and immunoelectrophoresis

Pamela G. Riches

1.1 INTRODUCTION   3

1.2 SUPPORT MEDIA FOR ELECTROPHORESIS   4
    1.2.1 *Clinical applications of electrophoresis*   5
    1.2.2 *Visualization of electrophoretic patterns*   6

1.3 IMMUNOELECTROPHORESIS   7
    1.3.1 *Classical immunoelectrophoresis*   8
    1.3.2 *Countercurrent immunoelectrophoresis*   9
    1.3.3 *Two-dimensional immunoelectrophoresis*   10
    1.3.4 *Transfer immunoelectrophoresis*   10
    1.3.5 *Immunofixation electrophoresis*   10

1.1 INTRODUCTION

For a detailed consideration of electrophoretic techniques and the factors which influence them the standard texts are recommended[1-3]. This discussion will be restricted to those aspects of electrophoresis which are most likely to affect the practical applications particularly as applied to proteins.

The charged groups of protein molecules are zwitterions and the net charge is strongly influenced by the pH of the buffer. As alkaline pH proteins behave entirely as anions whereas in acid conditions they are present as cations. There is a characteristic pH for each protein, its isoelectric point, at which it does not migrate since oppositely charged sites are balanced. It is also the point of minimum solubility of the protein. The mobility is, therefore, pH dependent although this is further modified by electroendosmosis. Buffers with a pH at or near the isoelectric point of relevant proteins must be avoided. The ionic strength of buffers influences the time taken for proteins to migrate over a given distance so that the more concentrated the buffer the slower will be the migration although zones are found to be sharper.

Zone electrophoresis is performed on a support medium. The supporting medium can affect the conditions of electrophoresis and hence influence separations. The charge effect of the support media causes some interaction with macromolecules and this together with variation in the amounts of electroendosmosis causes differences in comparative patterns obtained.

Electro-endosmosis is set up due to a net negative charge on the ions of the supporting medium. There is thus a tendency for these ions to move towards the anode, i.e. in the opposite direction to the electrophoretic flow; however, as these charged groups are immobilized in the support medium, a compensatory flow of buffer ions towards the cathode is set up sweeping with it more weakly charged protein ions. The net mobility of a charged particle is therefore the result of the movement due to charge and the resistance offered by the buffer flow due to electroendosmosis. If we consider serum proteins migrating at, e.g. pH 8.6 (barbitone buffer), the strongly charged anions such as albumin will move readily towards the anode whereas weakly charged molecules (such as γ-globulins) will be affected principally by electro-endosmosis and will be drawn towards the cathode.

1.2　SUPPORT MEDIA FOR ELECTROPHORESIS

For practical purposes in the routine clinical laboratory there are two main categories of support media in use.

(a) Cellulose acetate, agar and agarose. All are used with equal success for electrophoretic separations. They can be regarded as relatively inert with large pore sizes which do not hinder particle migration. The extent of electroendosmosis varies with the medium. Cellulose acetate and agar both show the property of high electroendosmosis. Agarose is now commercially available, from several sources, with a wide range of electroendosmosis varying from very low to very high. The degree of electroendosmosis should be selected to suit the separation.

(b) Starch and acrylamide gels have pore sizes of the same order of magnitude as protein molecules with the result that a molecular sieving effect is superimposed on the electrophoretic separation due to charge distribution. The patterns obtained on these media are more complex than those obtained with cellulose acetate (CAM), agar or agarose.

1.2.1 Clinical applications of electrophoresis

Electrophoresis on cellulose acetate or agarose should be performed in every case in which the plasma protein pattern may be expected to yield useful clinical information. It is essential for the diagnosis of paraproteinaemias and some congenital plasma protein aberrations.

The clinical situations in which protein electrophoresis has been found to be most useful are summarized in Table 1.1.

Electrophoretic separation of plasma proteins followed by visual inspection is a most valuable and informative procedure provided that a good, correctly

TABLE 1.1 Summary of clinical situations in which serum electrophoresis is indicated

---

1. Absolute indication, essential to diagnosis.
   No other procedure will provide same information as quickly or as economically.
      paraproteinaemias (myeloma, etc.)
      deficiency proteinaemias (agammaglobulinaemia, etc.)
      haemoglobinopathies
      some genetic aberrations (e.g. bisalbuminaemia, analbuminaemia, α_1-antitrypsin variants)
2. Clinically helpful indication in combination with other investigations.
      liver disease
      nephrotic syndrome
      malignancy
      collagen disease
3. Monitoring and management of disease in which significant alterations of serum protein occur.
   Valuable if same technique is used. Reliable results can be obtained even if not strictly correct in absolute terms,
      e.g. albumin
         abnormal protein in myeloma, etc.
4. Screening. Can be most valuable in population surveys for presence of abnormal proteins and for detection of inborn or acquired deficiencies.
      (e.g. α_1-antitrypsin, haemoglobins)

---

performed technique is employed. Separation should be of sufficient length to separate clearly the five major fractions – albumin, α_1, α_2, β and γ and also the minor prealbumin zone. Poor technique was responsible over many years for the neglect of prealbumin which can be a valuable marker in the assessment of clinical conditions.

Quantitative electrophoresis is only required for the estimation of monoclonal bands, that is paraproteins, that cannot be assayed reliably by immunochemical techniques. The protein content of each of the separated fractions comprises the sum total of all the constituent individual proteins which have only the same or similar electrophoretic migration. These proteins do, however, vary widely in their physical and biological properties. Consequently fraction quantitation by scanning or elution, even by the more sophisticated techniques, is of debatable value.

With the advent of reliable methods for quantitation of individual proteins there is no longer a valid justification for fraction quantitation unless that fraction is homogeneous.

Visual inspection of electrophoretic separations is recommended for recognition of characteristic patterns, some examples of which are illustrated in Table 1.2. It must be re-emphasized that these patterns are not pathognomonic but should be regarded rather as 'suggestive evidence'. These patterns are usually associated with more advanced stages of disease.

1.2.2   Visualization of electrophoretic patterns

A wide variety of techniques is available to demonstrate the separation pattern.

(1) Direct visualization by means of ultraviolet or infrared radiation.

(2) Precipitation by a non-specific agent followed by a staining procedure[4].

(3) Specific enzyme–substrate reactions resulting in the formation of coloured insoluble reaction products, e.g. for the detection of isoenzymes[5].

(4) Precipitation of macromolecules by specific antibodies. The resulting insoluble precipitate can be inspected directly or subsequently stained with suitable stains. This latter reaction forms the basis of the immunoelectrophoretic techniques. It can, therefore, be appreciated that electrophoresis and immunoelectrophoresis are two applications of the same basic principle of zone electrophoresis.

TABLE 1.2 Some examples of 'suggestive' protein electrophoretic patterns in disease

Prealbumin	Albumin	α_1	α_2	β	γ	Suggested disease
↓	↓	↑	N or ↑	N	N or ↓	Malignancy
↓↓	↓↓	Low N	Low N	N	↑↑↑	Cirrhosis of the liver
	↓↓	N	↑↑	N or ↑	↓	Nephrotic syndrome
N or ↓	↓	↑	↑	N	N	Acute infections
N or ↓	↓	N	↑	N	↑	Chronic infections
↓	↓	N	↑	N	↑ or ↑↑	Collagen diseases

N = Normal
↓ = Low
↑ = High

1.3 IMMUNOELECTROPHORESIS

Immunoelectrophoresis is a two-step procedure by which macromolecules (usually proteins) are first separated by zone electrophoresis and then subsequently reacted with appropriate antisera in the support medium. A wide variety of techniques is available for effecting the second step, some of which are considered below.

1.3.1   Classical immunoelectrophoresis

This technique was developed by Grabar and Williams in 1953[6]. Figure 1.1 illustrates the principle of this technique in which proteins are first separated, usually in buffered agar or agarose gel, and then lateral slots are cut at right angles alongside the separated components and filled with the required antisera. The separated proteins and the antisera are then left to diffuse (usually overnight) resulting in precipitation arcs formed by reaction between corresponding antigen and antibody.

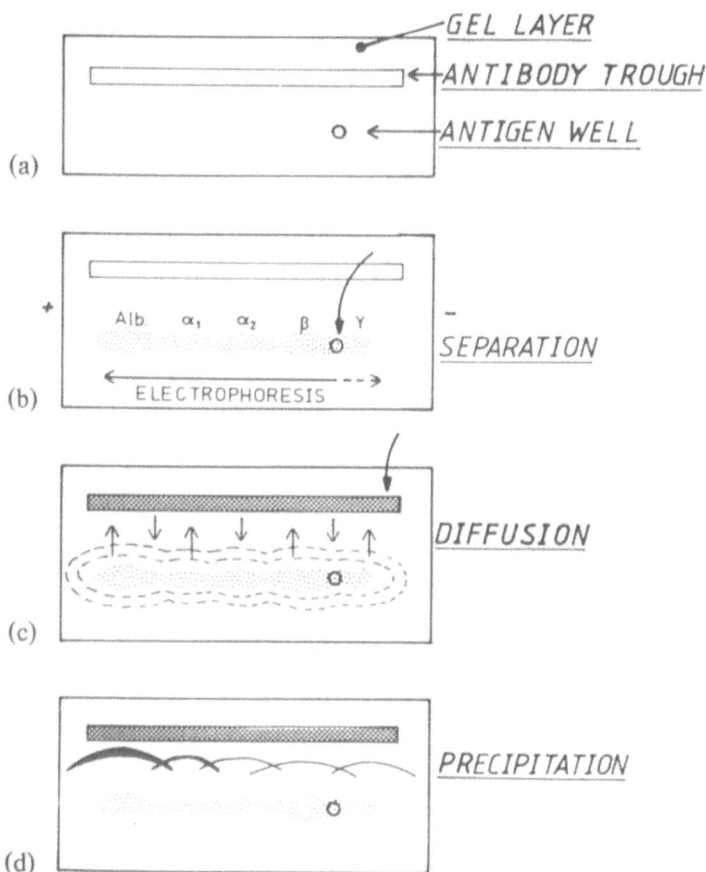

Figure 1.1   Principle of immunoelectrophoresis. Serum sample applied to well (a) is separated by zone electrophoresis into the major fraction, (b) antiserum is then applied into a trough (c) and diffusion of antigen and antibody into the support medium results in precipitation lines (d)

The principal application of immunoelectrophoresis is in demonstrating the antigenic pattern of a complex mixture of proteins and identifying individual proteins by the use of monospecific antisera. In the routine clinical laboratory immunoelectrophoresis is most usually applied to the typing of paraproteins in serum and to Bence Jones protein in serum or urine. Immunoelectrophoresis is not a quantitative technique.

1.3.2 Countercurrent immunoelectrophoresis

The principle of countercurrent immunoelectrophoresis is illustrated in Figure 1.2. The support medium can be agar, agarose or cellulose acetate[7]. Antibodies are immunoglobulins and at alkaline pH move cathodally due to electroendosmosis. If an antibody is placed on the anodal side of an antigen with anodic mobility then during electrophoresis the antigen and antibody will move towards each other resulting in precipitation at or near equivalence. Countercurrent immunoelectrophoresis can be used for the detection and identification of a wide range of proteins and other substances. The only limitation is that the antigen must have a mobility different from that of the antibody.

Countercurrent immunoelectrophoresis is very sensitive as all the antigens and antibodies move as a narrow zone giving maximum concentration for

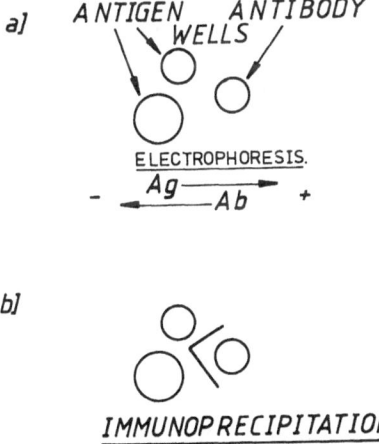

Figure 1.2 Principle of countercurrent immunoelectrophoresis. Antigen is applied cathodally to the appropriate antibody (a) and after electrophoresis a precipitation line can be seen (b)

reaction. It is also a very rapid technique ($1\frac{1}{2}$ hours from start to finish on cellulose acetate) and is, therefore, ideal as a screening test. Dissolution of precipitates in antigen excess can be avoided by the use of two antigen volumes (see Figure 1.2) or dilutions.

The specificity of a sample can also be checked by using two antigen wells of equal size; in one is placed a known antigen and into the second the unknown specimen. A fused line is confirmation of antigen identity.

1.3.3   Two-dimensional immunoelectrophoresis

Two-dimensional (or crossed) immunoelectrophoresis is a technique in which macromolecules separated by zone electrophoresis (usually on agarose gel) are electrophoresed into a second antibody containing gel at right angles to the first electrophoretic separation. Movement of proteins in the second dimension results in precipitation peaks. The area enclosed by each peak is proportional to the antigen:antibody ratio. The method can, therefore, be used for the simultaneous quantitation of a number of proteins in a complex mixture. It is also useful for studying protein heterogeneity, polymorphism, fragmentation and aggregation. It is used in the routine laboratory for studying complement breakdown products[8].

1.3.4   Transfer immunoelectrophoresis

This technique is a variant of the classical Grabar and Williams method, based on the same principle except that the initial electrophoretic separation is carried out on cellulose acetate[9]. The cellulose acetate is then transferred to the surface of an agar plate and filter paper strips impregnated with the required antiserum are placed about 3–5 mm away, parallel to the run. Antigens and antibodies diffuse into the agar and form precipitation arcs. An advantage over classical immunoelectrophoresis is that any fraction can be cut out and the antigenic pattern studied in isolation. This results in a much easier identification of individual proteins, particularly paraproteins, as the precipitation arcs are less crowded. A direct comparison of antigenic identity with the electrophoretic mobility on cellulose acetate is also possible.

1.3.5   Immunofixation electrophoresis

In immunofixation techniques electrophoretically separated proteins are reacted with appropriate antisera.

This method combines the speed and simplicity of electrophoresis with a rapid antigenic identification of individual proteins in a complex mixture. A parallel stained pattern provides the localization of the antigen. It is hoped that immunofixation will become a valuable technique in the routine laboratory. As this is a relatively recent development of immunoelectrophoresis and has not yet been described in the standard textbooks a more detailed account is required.

The term 'immunofixation' electrophoresis was first used by Alper and Johnson[10] in 1969. In this technique a protein-containing gel, after electrophoresis, is exposed to specific antisera. In an even earlier technique (Afonso, 1964)[11] combining electrophoresis with the principle of radial immunodiffusion, antiserum was layered on top of the separation pattern on agar gel, resulting in precipitation rings which were then quantitated.

Recently more modifications of these 'immunofixation' methods on agarose have been described[12]. The method has also been used for the phenotyping of α_1-antitrypsin at acid and alkaline pII[13], for the study of monoclonal bands in serum[14] and in cerebrospinal fluid[15] and for the phenotyping of the Gc-protein[16] which has also been reported using cellogel as the supporting medium[17].

An immunofixation method carried out entirely on CAM for locating and identifying individual proteins in biological fluids using specific antibody, however, is recommended for routine use[18]. This technique has all the advantages of the agarose system in terms of sensitivity, exact location of minor monoclonal bands and high resolution, with the added advantage of extreme speed and simplicity.

Electrophoresis is first carried out on CAM using fresh 6 mmol/l barbitone buffer pH 8.6 at a constant current of 0.4 mA/cm width as for routine electrophoresis, preferably on sheets 150×78 mm using a multiapplicator.

Antisera are diluted in buffer (as above) containing polyethylene glycol (PEG) at a final concentration of 4%. The required dilution depends on the titre, avidity and type of antiserum as well as the amount of antigen applied. Immunofixation is best done near equivalence of antigen and antibody. Excess antigen, for instance, causes dissolution in areas of highest antigen concentration, resulting in 'fixed' bands with unstained centres.

Antisera can be used at 10% of the initial concentration, and the protein band to be immunofixed is then diluted into the range 0.05–0.2 g/l. For more intense precipitation bands the protein is diluted into the range 0.5–1.0 g/l and the antiserum concentration is adjusted to 50%. All antisera should be filtered through 0.2 μm cellulose membrane filters after required dilution and before use. This is most important as it almost completely eliminates background staining. Diluted antisera can be re-used many times, although an occasional re-filter may be required.

Immediately after electrophoresis, the CAM is cut into appropriate segments which are then immersed for 5 minutes in antiserum kept in a suitable flat container. The strip is then rinsed off in running tap water and washed for 30 minutes in barbitone buffer (as for electrophoresis) containing 0.1% Triton X-100.

The staining procedure depends on the intensity of the antigen–antibody complex. The dense precipitate resulting from immunofixation in 50% diluted antisera can be detected by staining in 0.2% Ponceau S in 3% TCA. The less intense precipitate formed in 10% diluted antisera is better detected with a more sensitive stain. 0.1% Nigrosin in 5% acetic acid is used. The CAM segments are stained in the Nigrosin solution for 30 minutes followed by washing in tap water.

Figure 1.3 shows an IgG λ monoclonal band identified by immunofixation in 50% dilution of anti-IgG and anti-λ light-chain antisera. The combination of routine staining and immunofixation enables exact location of the paraprotein band. In this particular serum, immunofixation indicated that the band in the fast γ region, which could have been mistaken on routine electrophoresis for complement, was in fact a Bence Jones protein in the same position as the Bence Jones in the urine.

Figure 1.4 shows a series of urines stained before and after immunofixation to show the identity of the Bence Jones protein. The total amount of protein in these urines was 0.5–1.0 g/l.

Apart from the routine identification of paraprotein bands immunofixation on CAM has proved invaluable in several areas where previously there were difficulties in localization and/or identification. In particular:

(1) For identification of low concentrations of a paraprotein (in the region of 1 g/l), particularly in the presence of normal levels of immunoglobulins.

(2) For localization of paraproteins 'hidden' by other serum proteins, for example, IgA paraproteins masked by the α_2 and β regions.

(3) Detection and identification of Bence Jones proteins in serum.

(4) Identification of more than one paraprotein in serum.

(5) Light-chain typing of IgM paraproteins which is not always easy by immunoelectrophoresis and frequently involves reduction of the molecule to enable successful typing.

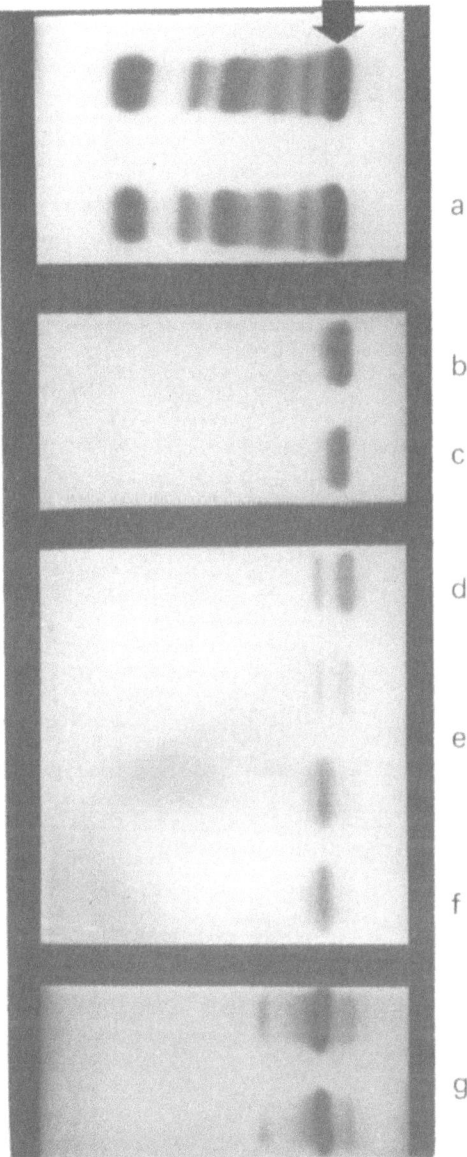

Figure 1.3 Identification and localization of a paraprotein (34 g/l) in serum and Bence Jones in the urine of a myeloma patient. Direct Ponceau S staining reveals a paraprotein in the γ region indicated by arrow (a). Serum diluted 1:50 (b), (d) and 1:100 (c, e) stained after immunofixation with anti-IgG (b, c) and anti-λ light-chains (d, e). The more anodic band seen in (d) and (e) is the Bence Jones protein also present in the urine (f). Nigrosin staining of the urine proteins (g) without immunofixation. Note only specific protein bands staining after immunofixation

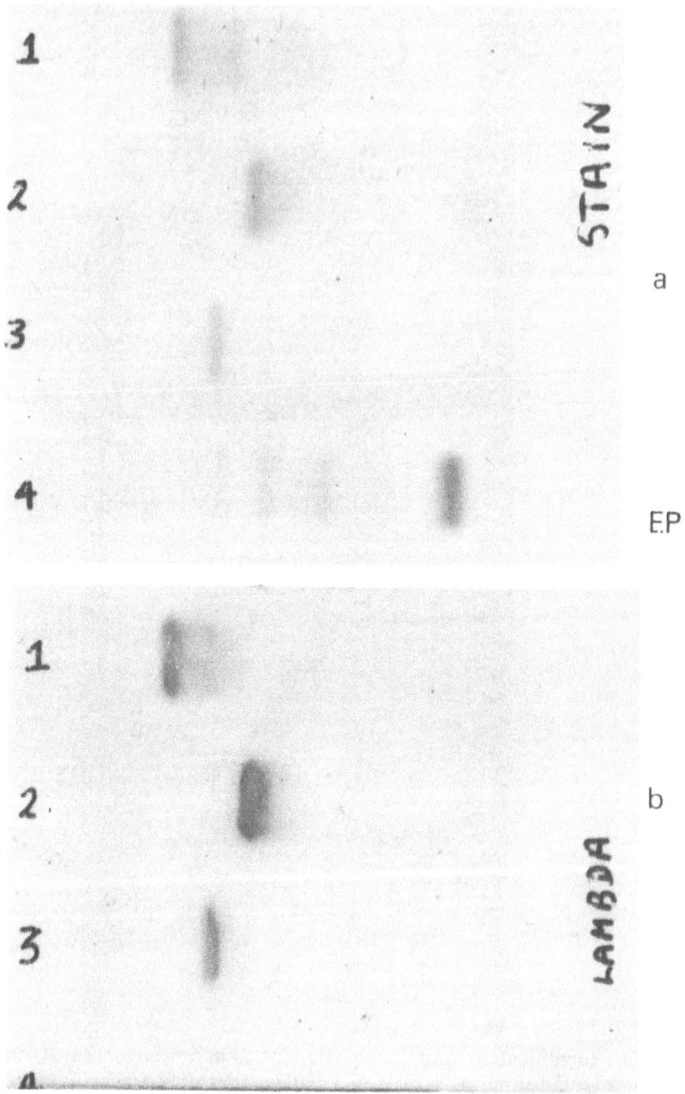

Figure 1.4 Identification of Bence Jones protein in urine by Ponceau S staining (a) and confirmation after immunofixation (b). Serum electrophoresis (EP) for orientation purposes

References

1. Cawley, L. P. (1969). *Electrophoresis and Immunoelectrophoresis*. (Boston: Little, Brown and Company)
2. Smith, I. (ed.) (1976). *Chromatographic and Electrophoretic Techniques*. Vol. II. (London: Heinemann)
3. Sargent, J. R. and George, S. G. (1975). *Methods in Zone Electrophoresis*. (Poole: BDH Chemicals Ltd.)
4. Kohn, J. (1976). Cellulose acetate electrophoresis and immuno-diffusion techniques. In: Ivor Smith (ed.). *Chromatographic and Electrophoretic Techniques*. Vol. II, pp. 102–112. (London: Heinemann)
5. Sciliano, M. J. and Shaw, C. R. (1976). Separation and visualization of enzymes on gels. In: Ivor Smith (ed.). *Chromatographic and Electrophoretic Techniques*, Vol. II, pp. 185–209. (London: Heinemann)
6. Grabar, P. and Williams, C. A. (1953). Methode permettant l'étude conjugée des propriétés electrophorétiques et immunochimiques d'un mélange de proteines. Application au serum sanguin. *Biochim. Biophys. Acta*, **10**, 193
7. Kohn, J. and Kahan, M. (1976). Countercurrent immunoelectrophoresis on cellulose acetate. *J. Immunol. Meth.*, **11**, 303
8. Versey, J. (1976). Quantitative immunoelectrophoresis. In: Ivor Smith (ed.). *Chromatographic and Electrophoretic Techniques*, Vol. II, pp. 347–366. (London: Heinemann)
9. Kohn, J. (1976). Cellulose acetate electrophoresis and immunoelectrophoresis. In: Ivor Smith (ed.). *Chromatographic and Electrophoretic Techniques*. Vol. II, pp. 120–126. (London: Heinemann)
10. Alper, C. A. and Johnson, A. M. (1969). Immunofixation electrophoresis: A technique for the study of protein polymorphism. *Vox Sang.*, **17**, 445
11. Afonso, E. (1964). Quantitative immunoelectrophoresis of serum proteins. *Clin. Chim. Acta*, **10**, 114
12. Ritchie, R. F. and Smith, R. (1976). Immunofixation: I. General principles and application to agarose gel electrophoresis. *Clin. Chim. Acta*, **22**, 497
13. Ritchie, R. F. and Smith, R. (1976). Immunofixation: II. Application to typing of α_1-antitrypsin at acid pH. *Clin. Chim. Acta*, **22**, 1735
14. Ritchie, R. F. and Smith, R. (1976). Immunofixation: III. Application to the study of monoclonal proteins. *Clin. Chim. Acta*, **22**, 1982
15. Cawley, L., Minard, B. J., Tourelotte, W. W., Ma., B.I. and Chelle, C. (1976). Immunofixation electrophoretic techniques applied to identification of proteins in serum and cerebrospinal fluid. *Clin. Chim. Acta*, **22**, 1262
16. Johnson, A. M., Cleve, H. and Alper, C. (1975). Variants of the group-specific component system as demonstrated by immunofixation electrophoresis. *Am. J. Hum. Genet.*, **27**, 728
17. Martin, W. and Voss, C. (1977). Gc-Immunofixation auf Cellogel-Folien. *Artztl. Lab.*, **23**, 337
18. Kohn, J. and Riches, P. (1978). A cellulose acetate immunofixation technique. *J. Immunol. Meth.*, **20**, 325

2

Radial immunodiffusion and rocket immunoelectrophoresis

D. Kenny

2.1 INTRODUCTION   17

2.2 PRINCIPLES   18

2.3 PRACTICAL DETAILS   19

2.4 MEASUREMENT OF PRECIPITATES   19

2.5 INFLUENCE OF MOLECULAR SIZE   20

2.6 ELECTROENDOSMOSIS AND ROCKET
     IMMUNOELECTROPHORESIS   21

2.1 INTRODUCTION

Specific protein concentrations may be measured in gel media by two techniques: single radial immunodiffusion and rocket immunoelectrophoresis. The former method is called 'single' to distinguish it from the qualitative Ouchterlony or 'double diffusion' methods, and 'radial' to contrast it with the earlier 'linear diffusion' technique of Oudin[1]. Rocket immunoelectrophoresis is also called 'electroimmunoassay'. The original versions of these techniques were described respectively by Mancini, Carbonara and Heremans in 1965[2], and Laurell in 1966[3]. Verbruggen[4] has recently published an extensive review of quantitative immunoelectrophoretic methods.

2.2 PRINCIPLES

In both methods antigen solutions are placed in wells punched in a flat gel layer which is of uniform thickness and contains a uniform concentration of specific antiserum. The antigen is then allowed to diffuse into the gel (in radial immunodiffusion) or is moved into it by the application of an electrophoretic field (in the rocket technique). As antigen advances it forms soluble complexes under conditions of antigen excess while at the leading edge antigen concentration is lower than in the body of the advancing sample and insoluble complexes are precipitated. As diffusion or electrophoresis proceeds the bonds between antigen and antibody are continuously broken and reformed, and the advancing free antigen redissolves the precipitate at the leading edge. This process continues until all free antigen is consumed and the precipitate is stationary since there is nothing available to redissolve it.

In radial immunodiffusion all directions receive equal doses of antigen and the final precipitate is ring-shaped.

In the rocket technique antigen is moved in one direction only and its concentration at the sides of this 'track' is soon reduced to that which forms a stable precipitate. This forms the sides of the 'rocket'; as the antigen moves further from the well and its concentration in the centre of the track is reduced the sides converge. When they meet in a point the final position has been reached.

Why is the precipitate not then dissolved by diffusion of excess antibody from the outside of the ring or rocket?

(a) It appears[5] that these precipitates form while the antigen is still in excess by the standards of the classical test-tube precipitation reaction, i.e. the final position of ring or rocket is reached before the antigen concentration has been reduced to the classical equivalence point, and the precipitates formed have a higher ratio of antigen to antibody than those found in tube experiments. It follows that the diffusion of further antibody into the region of these insoluble complexes brings conditions closer to equivalence and can intensify the precipitate.

(b) Such a dissolution might happen eventually with a plate containing horse antibodies, whose complexes tend to be soluble at both antigen and antibody excess, but the rabbit and goat antisera usually used for these techniques form soluble complexes at antigen excess only.

2.3 PRACTICAL DETAILS

It is not intended to give here the full details of procedures which are very well described in existing publications[2,6,7], but to draw attention to some practical points of importance and in particular to differences between the original methods and some widely used modifications.

In both of the original techniques the gels were cast between two glass plates separated by a U-shaped frame. Pouring the molten agarose onto a glass plate placed on a level surface is, with some practice, a quicker and less laborious technique. The lip of the tube from which the hot solution has just been poured is used to encourage rapid spreading. This method can be used successfully to produce plates of up to 20×10 cm in size. With the appropriate antiserum concentration and number of wells these plates are equally suitable for both rocket and radial immunodiffusion techniques.

In the rocket technique, electrical connection between the antibody-containing gel and the buffer vessels may be made through wicks made of paper or other absorbent material soaked in buffer solution, or through agarose gel bridges and connecting strips. Gel connections give more reliable contact, and the bridges although laborious to make can be re-used indefinitely provided that strips of dialysis membrane are used to prevent contamination with protein from the running gel.

Laurell's original paper recommends the use of barbitone buffer at a concentration of 75 mmol/l and voltages of up to 20 V/cm. Most other workers use lower voltages and buffer concentrations; 20 mmol/l barbitone and 2 V/cm are satisfactory for overnight running[6]. Even at such low voltages it is advisable to cool the plate with circulating water.

For the removal of non-precipitated proteins after the run, Laurell's technique of pressing the gel under wet filter paper is extremely effective. The use of prolonged washes in a saline bath is rarely necessary.

2.4 MEASUREMENT OF PRECIPITATES

In both techniques quantitation is based on the assumption that the area within the final precipitation line is a measure of the quantity of antibody consumed and is therefore proportional to the quantity of antigen placed in the well. A set of reference sera with assigned concentration values is assayed with the test samples and used to draw a standard curve from which the concentrations of test samples are determined. For best precision and accuracy a full standard curve as well as control sera should be run on each plate. Measuring areas directly is difficult, so that various indirect approaches are used. Mancini, Carbonara and Heremans in the original radial immunodiffusion technique[2] projected the rings on to paper, traced the outlines, and cut out and weighed the paper circles. They then expressed the size of the rings as milligrams of paper. This was intended to avoid the errors which would result from measuring the diameters of irregularly shaped rings. A simpler approach is to make duplicate measurements of the diameter at right angles and to reject irregular rings as unsuitable for measurement. The squares of the diameters are proportional to area and give a straight line plot against concentration, which is desirable since the interpolation of test readings on a non-linear standard curve is more open to error. The knowledge that the standard curve should be a straight also provides a good quality control check. Plotting the diameters (not squared) against concentration is sometimes done. This is not to be recommended since it amounts to throwing away the advantages of a linear standard curve for a very small saving in labour.

Measuring ring diameters while some of them are still growing gives non-linear and irreproducible standard curves on which interpolations are largely guesswork. The supposed relationship between log concentration and ring diameter is derived from a different technique (the linear diffusion method of Oudin[1]) and does not really apply in this situation. Such measurements can of course be used to obtain preliminary semiquantitative results when needed.

The measurement of rocket precipitates gives rise to some problems. Laurell[3] used peak height measurement, and this is still almost universal. The standard curves obtained are however not generally linear. Area measurements give better results in this respect but paper tracing methods are laborious and calculations involving peak width measurements are affected by the large error in measuring such small distances. The best compromise is probably to use peak height measurements except where the paper cut-out technique seems to have definite advantages, as in measuring 'cigar-shaped IgG precipitates.

2.5   INFLUENCE OF MOLECULAR SIZE

In radial immunodiffusion it is commonly found that molecular size influences the end result, for example that IgM monomers form larger rings than IgM polymers for the same quantity of protein. This is easily explained in techniques using incomplete diffusion, since the smaller molecules move more quickly through the gel. Why, given sufficient time, does the large protein not travel as far as the small one? (The situation should not be confused with that, say, of intact C3 and C3 fragments. Fragments which lack some of the antigenic determinants of the parent molecule can be expected to diffuse farther since they react with a smaller proportion of the antibodies present in the gel.) It may be that when the 'leading edge' of antigen–antibody complex is moving very slowly it receives a significant contribution of antibody by diffusion from outside, with the result that the antigen meets more antibody than the area of diffusion would suggest. Alternatively, the antigen molecules because of their large size may need fewer antobodies to bind them into insoluble complexes.

Size heterogeneity does not affect the rocket immunoelectrophoresis technique to the same extent, though charge heterogeneity may do. Small molecules do, however, diffuse rapidly to give cigar-shaped rockets during long electrophoretic runs; small proteins should be run for 4–6 hours at 10 V/cm rather than for 16 hours at 2 V/cm.

2.6 ELECTROENDOSMOSIS AND ROCKET IMMUNOELECTROPHORESIS

In rocket immunoelectrophoresis 'an electrophoretic field induces migration of the antigens and antibodies'[3]. Although it is sometimes stated (e.g. Axelsen et al.[6], Verbruggen[4]) that the antibodies should not migrate during the run, a redistribution takes place with different antibody populations moving at different rates, or in opposite directions, in a manner determined by the pH and the electroendosmosis of the medium. At pH 8.6 in agarose of 'medium' electroendosmosis rabbit antibodies move toward both anode and cathode. This type of distribution is well illustrated by the cigar-shaped rather than rocket precipitates formed during electroimmunoassay of human IgG. When agarose of very low electroendosmosis is used, IgG forms anodal rockets with only slight cathodal precipitation, illustrating the fact that immobile antibodies are not necessary for the formation of rocket-shaped precipitates.

It is thus clear that antigens of similar isoelectric point to the antibody in the gel will migrate both anodally and cathodally; this may be overcome by altering the net charge of the antibody in the gel (carbamylation)[8] or of the antigen (formylation)[9].

References

1. Oudin, J. (1952). Specific precipitation in gels and its application to immuno-chemical analysis. *Methods Med. Res.*, **5**, 335
2. Mancini, G., Carbonara, A. O. and Heremans, J. F. (1965). Immunochemical quantitation of antigens by single radial immunodiffusion. *Immunochemistry*, **2**, 235
3. Laurell, C.-B. (1966). Quantitative estimation of proteins by electrophoresis in agarose gel containing antibodies. *Anal. Biochem.*, **15**, 45
4. Verbruggen, R. (1975). Quantitative immunoelectrophoretic methods: a literature survey. *Clin. Chem.*, **21**, 5
5. Harboe, N. and Ingild, A. (1973). Immunization, isolation of immunoglobulins, estimation of antibody titre. In ref. 5, p.161
6. Axelson, N. H., Krøll, J. and Weeke, B. (1973). *A Manual of Quantitative Immunoelectrophoresis*. (Oslo: Universitetsforlaget)
7. Laurell, C. B. (ed.) (1972). Electrophoretic and immunoelectrophoretic analysis of proteins. *Scand. J. Clin. Lab. Invest.*, **29**, suppl. 124
8. Weeke, B. (1968). Carbamylated human immunoglobulins tested by electro-phoresis in agarose and antibody-containing agarose. *Scand. J. Clin. Lab. Invest.*, **21**, 351
9. Slater, L. (1975). IgG, IgA and IgM by formylated rocket immunoelectrophoresis. *Ann. Clin. Biochem.*, **12**, 19

3

Automated immunoprecipitation and laser nephelometry

P. A. E. White and R. Strong

3.1   HISTORICAL INTRODUCTION   23

3.2   AUTOMATED IMMUNOPRECIPITATION   24
      3.2.1   *Fluoronephelometer*   24
      3.2.2   *Methodology*   25
      3.2.3   *Antigen–antibody concentration and antigen excess* 26

3.3   LASER NEPHELOMETRY   28
      3.3.1   *Optics of the laser nephelometer*   29
      3.3.2   *Methodology*   30

3.4   CORRELATIONS OF ESTIMATIONS BETWEEN
      METHODS   31

3.1   HISTORICAL INTRODUCTION

Quantitative determination of proteins by immunological methods began with the quantitative precipitin technique of Heidelberger and Kendall in 1935[1].

In 1938 Libby[2] combined immunology with nephelometry to measure the potency of antipneumococcal antiserum. In 1943 Boyden and Defalco[3] studied several immunoassay methods and concluded that light-scattering methods with low levels of reactants were superior to the quantitative precipitin analysis of Heidelberger.

In 1959 Schultze and Schwick[4] published the first clinically applicable methods for the immunoanalysis of several human plasma proteins. However, antiserum was scarce and of poor quality. In 1967 Ritchie[5] described a simple manual method for turbidimetric measurement of protein in dilute solution, the sensitivity of the technique having been increased with the use of high potency antibody to quantitate CSF immunoglobulins. Alper and Propp (1968)[6] applied nephelometry to the analysis of C3 and a year later Ritchie et al.[7] presented an improved, fully automated nephelometric system that was eventually refined further to become the Automated Immunoprecipitin (AIP) System marketed commercially by Technicon Instruments Corporation. A more rapid method developed by Larson et al.[8] for the Autoanalyser II system was based on the original Technicon AIP system which utilized polyethylene glycol (PEG) to accelerate the antigen–antibody reaction described in the work of Hellsing[9]. Sensitivity was increased, reaction time reduced and improved accuracy and ease of operation resulted. The PEG methodology has become the standard for the AIP system.

The use of a laser beam following the work of Blume and Greenberg[10] and Sieber and Gross[11] as a light source in nephelometric measurements has led to the development of the 'laser nephelometer'.

3.2   AUTOMATED IMMUNOPRECIPITATION

Nephelometry is the measuring of light scattered from particles suspended in a clear medium as opposed to turbidimetry which is defined as the measurement of light absorbed by suspended particles. Nephelometry measures the amount of light that has been reflected by the particles and therefore the density of the reactants must be much lower than for turbidimetry. In the AIP system the photoreceptor collects light reflected at 90° from the incident beam.

3.2.1   Fluoronephelometer

The wavelength for the incident light beam is based upon the size of the material in suspension and the light used in the Technicon Fluoronephelometer is an 85 watt mercury lamp. An optical filter is inserted into the light path so that only light at 355 nm can enter the flowcell. The light energy scattered from the particles is converted by a sample photomultiplier to an electric current that is proportional to the light energy striking the photomultiplier. The light energy is proportional to the scatter and is therefore a measure of concentration. The output of the fluoronephelometer is the result of a comparison between a reference photomultiplier, which is unaffected by material in the flowcell, and the output of the sample photomultiplier. This cancels out any effect on the recorder which may be caused by fluctuations in source lamp intensity.

3.2.2 Methodology

In the AIP system, specific antibody (antiserum) reacts with the specific protein to be analysed in dilute solution in antibody excess. The complexes formed are measured on a chart recorder from the signal from the fluoro-nephelometer. The basic antigen–antibody reaction follows the law of mass action in that the amount of complexes formed is a function of both antigen and antibody concentrations. The antibody concentration is kept constant while the antigen concentration is varied by using standards of known concentration and unknown test samples. The amount of complexes formed is therefore a function of the antigen concentration. In dilute solution these complexes remain in solution and their concentration is determined by measuring the light scattered at right angles to the incident beam. The amount of light scattered is a function of the number and molecular size of the complexes formed as well as the wavelength of light. Under test conditions the size of the molecules varies only slightly and so the amount of light scattered is proportional to the antigen concentration.

To accelerate the reaction the antibody can be diluted with 4% PEG solution in nephelometric-grade saline (particle-free normal saline + Tween 20).

Serum sample and saline are alternatively aspirated into the system at the rate of 120 samples/hour and diluted with nephelometric-grade saline (the amount of dilution being dependent upon the particular protein to be assayed) (Figure 3.1). The diluted sample is mixed in a six-turn coil and an aliquot of this introduced into a six-turn coil with the appropriate diluted and filtered antiserum. Complexes are formed in about 3 minutes and the amount of light scattered is measured by the fluoronephelometer and represented on the chart recorder as a series of peaks. Because of the inherent light-scattering properties of serum, a blank correction is usually required. The test run is repeated (both standards and samples) substituting 4% PEG–6000 saline for the antiserum

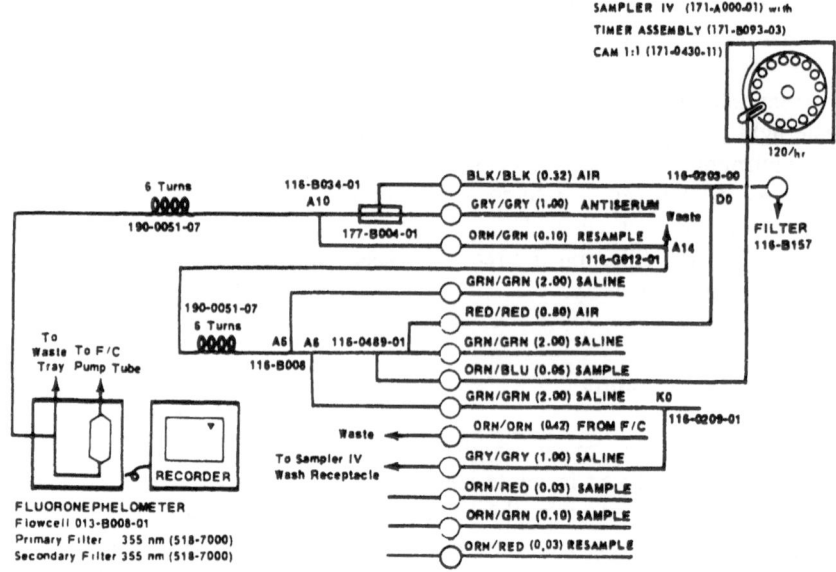

Figure 3.1 Flow diagram of AIP manifold as modified for the use of 48% poly-ethylene glycol (Reproduced by kind permission of Technician International Division, S.A.)

and subtracting the blank peak heights from their corresponding reaction peak heights (Figure 3.2).

3.2.3 Antigen–antibody concentration and antigen excess

Antigen and antiserum concentrations can be infinitely varied depending on the protein to be assayed and the potency of the antiserum (usual dilution of 1:60 to 1:80 in nephelometric-grade saline) by varying pump tube sizes on the manifold. For each protein assay a four- or five-point standard curve should be prepared using dilutions of a reference serum containing elevated levels of all proteins to be measured. The ratio of antigen to antibody in the system is devised so that each assay is linear within the normal range. By inserting an air bubble to eliminate laminar flow mixing of samples, each sample is subdivided into a series of individual subsamples, and a single test into multiple tests which are combined into a single peak on the recorder.

Samples containing very high concentrations of the protein being assayed can lead to an antigen excess condition. Owing to the early and late sub-

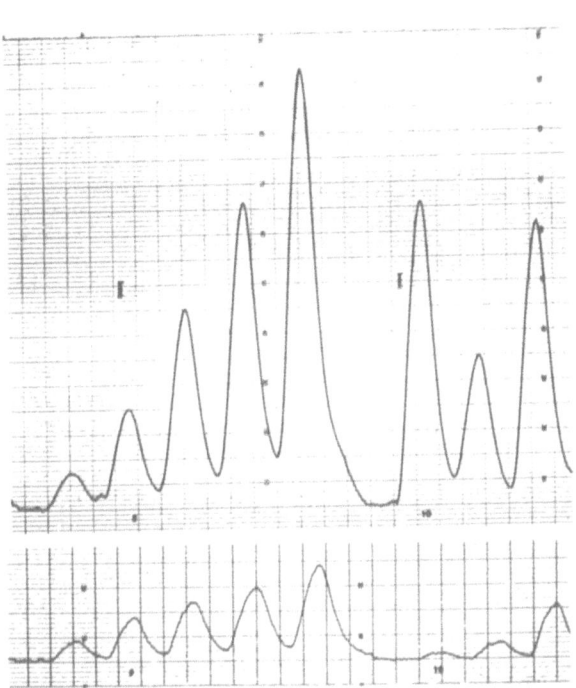

Figure 3.2 AIP analysis of human IgA showing reaction peaks from the chart recorder and their corresponding blank peaks below

samples being of low concentration the normal reaction occurs at the leading and trailing edges of the peak. Between these points soluble complexes are formed which result in a deflection of the chart recorder pen towards zero producing a 'twin peak' effect on the recorder (Figure 3.3). It can require considerable experience by the technologist to interpret these aberrant peak forms.

It is worth noting that it has been reported[12] that heparin plasma samples can produce extremely high 'false' blanks when using the PEG–6000 method. Adjustments in diluents can be made but it is not feasible to include heparin plasma samples and serum in the same run.

3.3 LASER NEPHELOMETRY

Laser is an acronym of Light Amplification by Stimulated Emission of Radiation.

The electronic signal from a nephelometer is highly dependent upon the light energy input from the incident beam. Because of the high light intensity that can be achieved in a monochromatic laser beam a substantial increase in sensitivity, and hence the ability to detect weak light scattering, can be achieved.

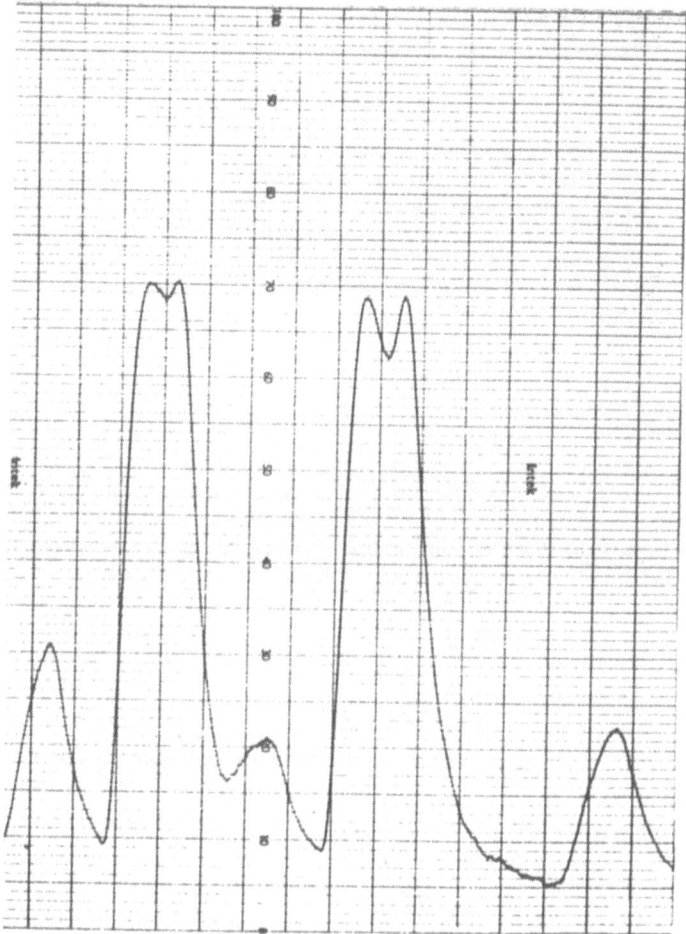

Figure 3.3 AIP analysis of human IgA illustrating the 'twin peak' effect of antigen excess in two samples of high concentration

The He–Ne laser consists of a slender glass plasma tube which surrounds a glass laser core and high energy pumping electrode. The glass plasma tube and core are filled with free helium and neon. A fully reflective mirror is positioned at the rear of the tube and a partially reflective mirror at the front. When the electrode is charged electrically, the He atoms are excited to a high energy state and by collision, transfer energy to the Ne atoms. The excited Ne atoms randomly emit photons. When interaction between these atoms occurs, the Ne atoms are now capable of amplifying light by stimulated emission. Many of the photons will bounce back and forth between the end mirrors many times, stimulating many other atoms to emit photons with each phase resulting in an amplification. Since one mirror is slightly transparent a portion of light bouncing between the mirrors will leak out, to produce the laser beam. Laser light has three major characteristics. It has high intensity, a high degree of collimation and is monochromatic.

3.3.1 Optics of the laser nephelometer

The intensity of the beam of scattered light is not measured at 90° to the incident beam as in the AIP system. The intensity of the scattered light is dependent on the angle between the incident beam and the axis on which the

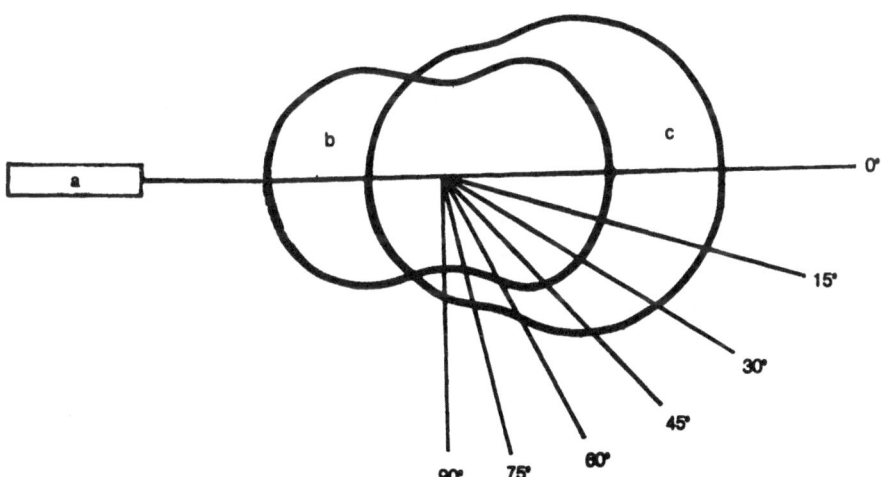

Figure 3.4 Angular dependence of light scattering as a function of particle geometry. (a) source (b) relative scattering envelope for small particles and (c) relative scattering envelope for large particles

photodetector is positioned. It has been known for many years that for large particles increases in scattering intensity can be obtained at angles less than 90°. According to Rayleigh[13], the intensity of scatter from a particle which is small relative to the wavelength should be symmetrically distributed about an axis which is at right angles to the incident beam.

However, for larger particles, whose dimensions approach the wavelength of light used for analysis, destructive interference of the light scattered from individual elements can occur resulting in a decrease in total scattering measured. Phase differences between scattered radiation, which cause the destructive interference, are reduced as the angle of observation approaches zero, resulting in an asymmetrical scattering envelope and significant angular dependence (Figure 3.4). In practice, the angle of observation is set between 30° and 35°.

The incident beam passes through the cell and is absorbed in a light trap. The cell holds the sample cuvette (thin walled plastic or glass) and the scattered light from the sample is detected and converted into an instrument reading.

3.3.2   Methodology

A series of dilutions of a standard serum is prepared together with dilutions of the test sera. To these the appropriate antisera are added. Because of the inherent light-scattering properties of serum a duplicate series of blanks must be prepared for each standard and test sample substituting saline or buffer for the antiserum. The antiserum solution itself is measured for its native light scattering ability. After mixing, each cuvette is incubated for 15 to 60 minutes and the cuvettes read. Each test reading of standard and sample has the antibody blank subtracted as well as its corresponding blank reading. The corrected readings of standards are plotted on a standard curve and the unknown sera concentrations calculated.

The ratio of signal to blank or noise is a problem and has been tackled in two ways. The most obvious way to minimise the blank is to remove the cause of it and this can be done by individually filtering each serum. This is expensive if cellulose acetate filters are used and is time consuming. The addition of dextran sulphate has been proposed but in some cases we have found the light scattering of the blank has actually increased after such a procedure. The second way to improve the signal to noise ratio is to enhance the signal in some way and this has been achieved by the use of PEG–4000. It is said that the addition of PEG to serum alone will increase the intensity of light scattered by causing a non-specific precipitation of protein. In the past this has not always been allowed for by incorporating PEG in the blank solution.

In one commercially available nephelometer the signal due to the scattered light is scanned continuously for between 5 and 90 seconds. The 'mean' signal is produced using solid state circuitry and the signal is filtered electronically to remove spikes caused by dust particles, etc. The instrument has also the facility to electronically subtract the antisera and serum blank readings from the test. The final reading obtained is therefore fully corrected for relevant blank values and is ready for plotting or reading off from the standard curve. Other nephelometers are also available using laser and non-laser light sources, and one employs reaction rate rather than end point measurement to assess light scatter.

3.4 CORRELATIONS OF ESTIMATIONS BETWEEN METHODS

Quantitations that are most frequently made are the immunoglobulins (IgG, IgA and IgM) together with albumin and C3. Disregarding minor differences all immunoglobulins have a unique physicochemical structure which leads to problems in their assessment since IgG, IgA and IgM tend to aggregate into discrete polymeric species. Within the normal range there is good correlation between RID and AIP value (Figure 3.5). There is also good correlation between results obtained by AIP and laser techniques; IgG, IgA, albumin and C3 are comparatively easily quantitated. IgM, however, gives more problems. Pathologically significant 7S forms of IgM exist either by themselves or more usually in varying amounts with the normal 19S component. The AIP system provides a direct measurement of the number of antigen–antibody complexes. In extreme cases a sample containing predominantly 7S molecules will produce very large diffusion rings by RID leading to a gross overestimate of IgM concentration. Conversely aggregated IgM samples diffuse more slowly by RID leading to underestimates.

There are similar quantitation ranges for AIP and laser techniques, both of which are rather better than for RID. There are, however, problems in quantitation of proteins with levels outside the normal range, i.e. very high or very low levels.

With RID very low levels give small diameter rings which can lead to small errors caused either by dilution or ring reading. These errors will produce large percentage errors in the final result. With high levels of protein there is the problem of the ring going to completion and the shape of the curve can make the result artificially high. With AIP and laser techniques the graph is more linear and offers a greater range of values. It is important to note that with the laser system antigen excess conditions are not as readily apparent as they are with the AIP system. Samples containing expectedly high levels of the

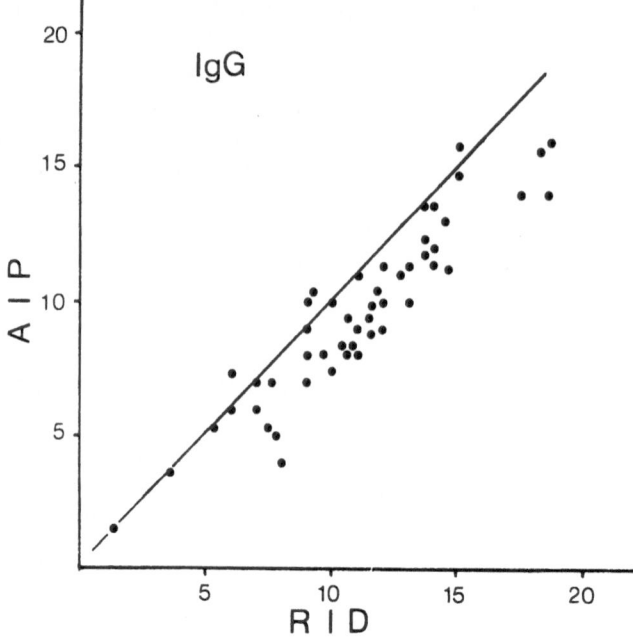

Figure 3.5 Comparison of results obtained for IgG using AIP and RID (units g/l)

protein to be assayed must be re-read after the addition of extra antigen; a reduction in light scattering indicates the antigen excess state and the sample must be reanalysed at dilution.

References

1. Heidelberger, M. and Kendall, F. E. (1935). Quantitative theory of precipitin reaction: study of cryoprotein:antibody system. *J. Exp. Med.*, **62**, 467
2. Libby, R. L. (1938). New and rapid quantitation technique for the determination of potency of types I and II antipneumococcal serum. *J. Immunol.*, **34**, 269
3. Boyden, A. and Defalco, R. J. (1943). Report on the use of the photron-reflectometer in serological comparisons. *Physiol. Zool.*, **16**, 229
4. Schultze, H. E. and Schwick, G. (1959). Quantitative immunologische Bestimmung von Plasmaproteinen. *Clin. Chim. Acta*, **4**, 15
5. Ritchie, R. F. (1967). A simple direct and sensitive technique for measurement of specific protein in dilute solution. *J. Lab. Clin. Med.*, **70**, 512
6. Alper, C. A. and Propp, R. P. J. (1968). Genetic polymorphism of the third component of complement (C3). *J. Clin. Invest.*, **47**, 2181

7. Ritchie, R. F., Alper, C. A. and Graves, J. A. (1969). Experience with a fully automated system of immunoassay of specific serum proteins (abstract). *Arthritis Rheum.*, **12,** 693

8. Larson, C., Gorman, J. M. and Becker, A. M. (1972). Automated immuno-precipitin system for proteins in body fluids − further advances. In: *Advances in Automated Analysis, Technicon International Congress,* Vol. 4, p.15. (Tarry-town, N.Y.: Mediad Inc. (1973))

9. Hellsing, K. (1972). Influence of polymer on the antigen−antibody reaction in a continuous flow system. In: *Automated Immunoprecipitin Reactions. Colloquium on AIP, Brussels* (ed. Technicon Instruments Corp.) p.17. (Tarrytown, N.Y.)

10. Blume, P. and Greenberg, L. (1975). Application of differential light scattering to the latex agglutination assay for rheumatoid factor. *Clin. Chem.,* **21/9,** 1234

11. Sieber, A. and Gross, J. (1975). Determination of proteins by laser nephelometry. *Protides of the Biological Fluids, 23rd Colloquium,* p. 295. (Oxford: Pergamon Press)

12. Shenkin, A., Morrison, B. and Robertson, D. A. (1977). Some problems in the correction for intrinsic light scattering of samples in specific protein analysis by automated immunoprecipitation. *Ann. Clin. Biochem.,* **14(3),** 163

13. Rayleigh, Lord (1871). On the scattering of light by small particles. *Philos. Mag.,* **12,** 81

4

Antiserum requirements
A. C. Munro

4.1 INTRODUCTION — 36

4.2 GENERAL FACTORS INVOLVED IN ANTISERUM
PRODUCTION — 36

4.3 IMMUNOGEN — 37
   4.3.1 *Origin, preparation and purification* — 37
   4.3.2 *Characterization* — 38

4.4. IMMUNIZATION — 39
   4.4.1 *Dose, adjuvant and protocol* — 39
   4.4.2 *Species and genetic variations* — 39

4.5 EVALUATION OF ANTISERA — 40
   4.5.1 *Specificity, titre and avidity* — 40
   4.5.2 *Suitability for individual test methods* — 42

4.2 PROCESSING — 45
   4.6.1 *Absorption* — 45
   4.6.2 *Fractionation* — 45
   4.6.3 *Additives and presentation* — 46

4.7 CONCLUSIONS — 48

4.1   INTRODUCTION

Developments in laboratory medicine and technology in recent years have greatly increased the demands for high quality animal antisera. The widespread use of antisera in immunochemical procedures and other techniques results from several unique properties possessed by these molecules. Firstly, they have the ability to detect single substances, ranging from high molecular weight proteins to low molecular weight drugs, in complex mixtures of closely related substances. Secondly, reactions involving antibodies are quantitative in nature and thirdly, these reactions may be made extremely sensitive and precise by the application of the appropriate methodology. However, the specificity, sensitivity and precision of immunochemical assays depend to a large extent on the intrinsic characteristics of the antibodies used.

Despite the widespread use of antisera as laboratory diagnostic reagents, their production and characterization are carried out largely on an empirical basis and there exist few general rules governing the production of antisera for specific laboratory methods. As a result the manufacturers of antisera, who are expected to produce uniform diagnostic reagents year after year, are confronted by very difficult standardization problems. It can be difficult to produce small amounts of antisera locally for an individual laboratory's needs; it is even more difficult to produce large volumes of high quality antisera which are to be used regionally, nationally or internationally, in a range of methods, by workers possessing no less a range of skills.

In 1971, an MRC Working Party on the clinical use of immunological reagents published a series of recommendations relating to the production and characterization of diagnostic antisera[1]. This represents one of the few attempts to define the area and the recommendations still hold good today. Indeed, with the introduction of more sophisticated and sensitive laboratory methods, these principles are all the more important. The remainder of this discussion will enlarge on these principles, with additional recommendations being made in some areas, and examples of various features will be drawn from our own experiences in antiserum production.

4.2   GENERAL FACTORS INVOLVED IN ANTISERUM
PRODUCTION

Any discussion of antiserum requirements should begin with a general consideration of the methods used for production. The processes involved can be broken down into several stages, as depicted in Figure 4.1. Firstly, a suitable immunogen, i.e. a substance which will stimulate the production of antibodies

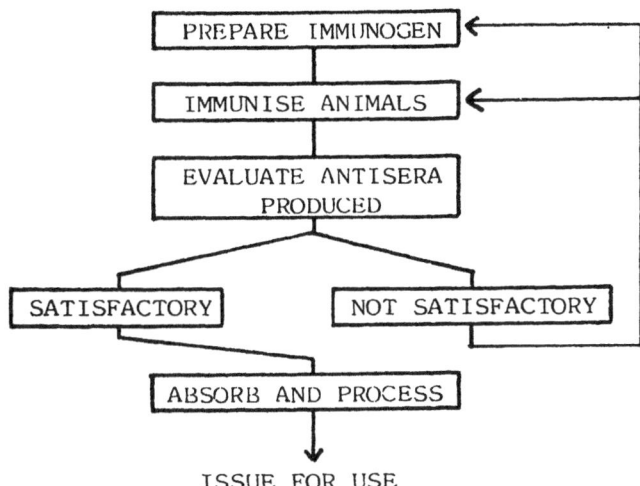

Figure 4.1 General method of antiserum production

when injected into animals must be prepared. In practice, immunogens are prepared in various forms or degrees of purity, depending on several factors including the nature of the tests in which the derived antisera will ultimately be used. The immunization process in animals presents several difficulties, not least of which is the unpredictability of the immune response in individual animals. Following the immunization of animals, antisera are evaluated and a choice of decisions is presented. Either the antisera are judged to be satisfactory in which case they will be further processed and issued or sold for use. If the antisera are unsuitable in any way the procedures used must be reconsidered and if necessary begun again with a new immunogen preparation, or by modifying the immunization protocol in a new group of animals.

4.3   IMMUNOGEN

4.3.1   Origin, preparation and purification

In order to induce an antibody response to drugs or low molecular weight hormones, the latter must usually be chemically linked to a protein to form a classical hapten–carrier conjugate. Some of the linking procedures commonly used are not completely reproducible and the chemical analysis of the resulting conjugate may be difficult, indeed in some cases impossible. It is therefore difficult to predict how immunogenic preparations of this type will be. However, with naturally-occurring protein immunogens, as are frequently measured in immunochemical techniques, this problem does not exist but is replaced by the requirement to purify the immunogen to a high degree prior to immunization. This reduces the possibility of antibodies of undesired specificities being produced. At the same time, extensive purification procedures increase the risk of degradation of labile serum proteins such as human IgM_2 and it can be difficult to purify some immunogens which normally occur in low concentrations, e.g. human IgE.

The origin of the immunogen should represent as closely as possible the normal variation encountered with this material. Immunoglobulin immunogens provide good examples of difficulties in this area. Whereas human IgG is relatively easy to isolate in a high degree of purity from normal human serum, the isolation of the other human immunoglobulins from the same source presents greater problems. In order to circumvent these problems some workers and presumably some manufacturers have used immunoglobulin immunogens isolated from myeloma sera, where they occur in high concentrations. Since the homogeneous myeloma proteins isolated are not entirely representative of the normal heterogeneous spectrum it is likely that antisera produced with these preparations will not react in identical fashion with all immunoglobulin molecules. A pool of monoclonal proteins is a possible alternative[1], although this may be difficult to acquire with IgD and almost impossible with IgE.

Another example of the problem of immunogen origin is seen with ferritin. In this case potential immunogens may be prepared from various sources and studies of this problem have indicated[3,4] that human liver is the preferred source for the subsequent production of anti-ferritin sera for use in determining serum ferritin levels.

4.3.2 Characterization

All protein immunogens should be rigorously characterized for immunochemical purity. For this purpose antisera which detect all possible impurities in the immunogen should be used. Since the immune system of an animal is a more sensitive indicator of purity than conventional immunochemical procedures, any impurities detected at this stage are almost certainly liable to induce the formation of unwanted antibody specificities.

A number of serum proteins are sensitive to the various precipitation, chromatography and ultracentrifugation procedures used in their purification. In our hands, human IgM has shown a remarkable propensity to break down into 7S and smaller fragments during purification and storage[2], even under the most carefully chosen conditions. It is suggested that the immunochemical characterization of immunogens should therefore be supplemented by physico-chemical analysis prior to immunization. For example, it is our practice to check the S values of preparations at this stage.

4.4 IMMUNIZATION

4.4.1 Dose, adjuvant and protocol

The immunization stage is probably subject to the greatest variation of all the stages in antiserum production. The dose of immunogen given can substantially affect the nature of the antibodies produced and, in general, the best antisera are obtained using small doses of material, in the range 10–100 μg for many human proteins. Small doses conserve valuable immunogen preparations and induce high titres of avid antibodies. In addition, there is a greater probability that small amounts of impurities not detectable by conventional immuno-chemical analysis will be presented to the animal below the threshold level of recognition for antibody stimulation.

In order to stimulate high levels of antibodies, immunogens are usually incorporated in an adjuvant, especially for the first (priming) injection. The most common form used is Freund's adjuvant, both in complete and incomplete forms, which present the immunogen in slow-release depots, in addition to non-specific stimulation of the animal's immune system. The protocol for immunization, i.e. the sequence, timing and route of injections, is undoubtedly important, although individual antibody producers have their own ideas in this area, based on past experience as to what is likely to succeed and what is not. Under normal circumstances it will require several weeks, months or even years before animals will produce good levels of suitable antibodies.

4.4.2 Species and genetic variations

Small animals such as rabbits are good antibody producers but in order to obtain good yields of antisera large colonies of animals must be maintained. Sheep and goats overcome this limitation by virtue of their larger size, and even larger volumes of antisera may be obtained from horses or donkeys, although the use of these animals involves increased costs and greater expertise in husbandry. Donkeys have been particularly successful for the production of second (precipitating) antisera for radioimmunoassays.

In general terms, the choice of species for optimum antibody response should reflect a high degree of foreignness of the immunogen. However, in some cases the best species for immunization defies rational explanation. In the case of antisera against the four sub-classes of human IgG, guinea pigs have been reported[5] as the best species for producing anti-IgG_1, and monkeys for producing anti-IgG_2 and anti-IgG_4.

Within any species a variation exists between individual animals in both the levels and characteristics of antibodies which can be induced. These variations would appear to reflect genetic differences between animals and there is therefore always an element of chance in the immune response. For example, Figure 4.2 illustrates the results obtained by immunizing a group of three sheep with purified human IgG. One animal produced high levels of antibodies in a short time, a second required several booster injections in order to acquire the same status, but the third never produced acceptable titres of suitable antibodies.

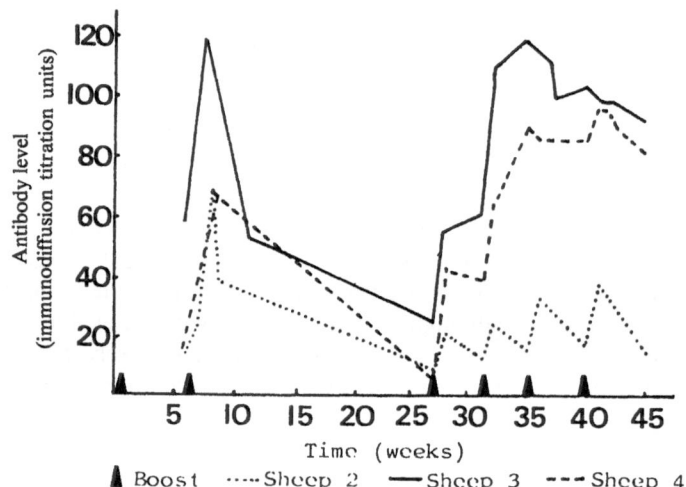

Figure 4.2 Immunization of sheep with purified human IgG (see Figure 4.4 for key to method)

4.5 EVALUATION OF ANTISERA

4.5.1 Specificity, titre and avidity

Generally, evaluations of antisera are carried out on small test bleeds taken from the animals. The assessment must be exact and rapid because antibody levels induced by booster injections of immunogens can rise and fall off in a matter of days, depending on the technique used.

With certain types of antisera, e.g. those used in competitive binding immunoassays, a high degree of specificity may not be important. Antibodies against carrier proteins or other unrelated substances may be tolerable in the final test situation. However in these cases the emphasis of purity shifts to the labelled steroid, protein or hormone used. With antisera for serological applications, e.g. Coombs reagents, it is difficult to define the specificity and there is no general agreement amongst workers as to which specificities are required[6]. However, for immunochemical applications specificity is of prime importance. Antisera should be demonstrated to react only with proteins representative of the appropriate types or classes used for immunization. The lack of complete specificity in these cases may be due to antibodies against unrelated proteins, arising through the use of an impure immunogen; alternatively, unwanted specificities may arise because of cross-reactivity between the immunogen and structurally related proteins. This is of course particularly evident with the immunoglobulins which share common light-chain determinants.

In two studies reported in 1970[7] and 1971[8], a large number of commercially available anti-human IgG, IgA and IgM sera were examined for specificity. Only 5% of the anti-IgG sera tested were shown to be specific for IgG and 25–33% of anti-IgA and anti-IgM sera were specific for these immunoglobulins. In some cases anti-IgM sera were specific for α_2-macroglobulin and not IgM itself. However, the position appears to be improving. The same workers reported more recently[9] on specificity studies of six manufacturers' IgG, IgA and IgM radial immunodiffusion plates. Whereas in 1973 only one of the six manufacturers' plates was shown to be immunoglobulin class-specific, by 1976 three out of six IgG, and all IgA and IgM plates, were shown to have acceptable specificity.

In our experience, and probably that of most antibody producers, tests of specificity of antisera removed from animals frequently demonstrate unwanted antibodies, despite the use of highly purified immunogens. Almost as important as the question of specificity then is the question of the ease of absorption of these unwanted specificities. Usually both of these points must be considered together when antisera are being assessed.

The titre and avidity of antisera should be of a high order. High titres, reflecting high antibody contents, ensure that antisera may be used at high dilutions, thus minimizing the possibility of interference effects by other serum proteins present. High avidities mean that the equilibrium of the antigen–antibody reaction is rapidly achieved, and that a high degree of binding between antigen and antibody ensues.

4.5.2   Suitability for individual test methods

It is essential that antisera are evaluated for their suitability for individual test methods. It does not follow that an antiserum which works well in one technique will necessarily work well in other techniques, even closely related ones. This is particularly apparent when comparing gel diffusion and nephelometric techniques where striking differences may be observed, despite the apparent similarities in the principles of both methods. Figure 4.3 depicts an example of this feature. Here a donkey was immunized with purified rabbit IgG and the levels of specific antibodies appearing during immunization were assessed by reversed single radial immunodiffusion, laser nephelometry and an immunodiffusion titration technique. Although all three methods show broadly similar results there are individual differences with certain bleeds, especially towards the end of the immunization course, where the nephelometric activity is particularly high.

Similar features may be observed in other species with different antisera. A series of bleeds from a sheep immunized with purified human IgG were tested in similar fashion to the above and the results obtained were subjected to regression analysis, as shown in Figures 4.4 and 4.5. A statistically

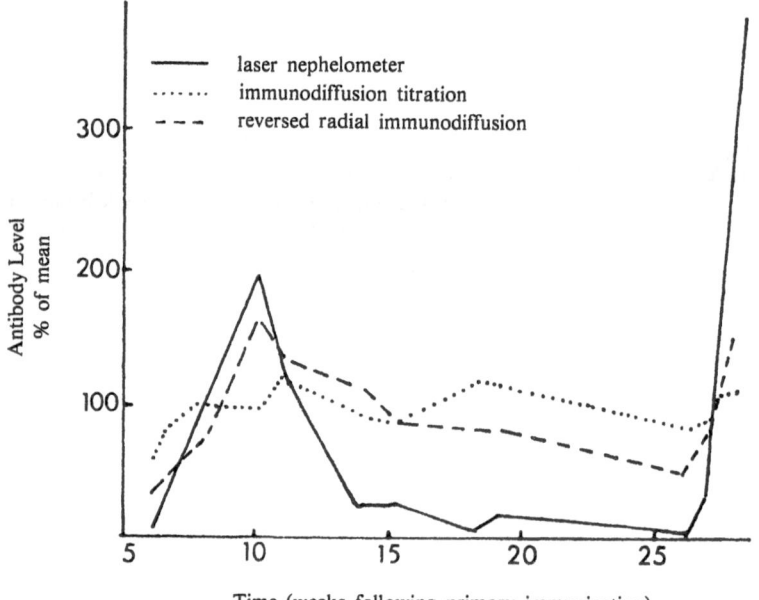

Figure 4.3   Immunization of donkey with purified rabbit IgG

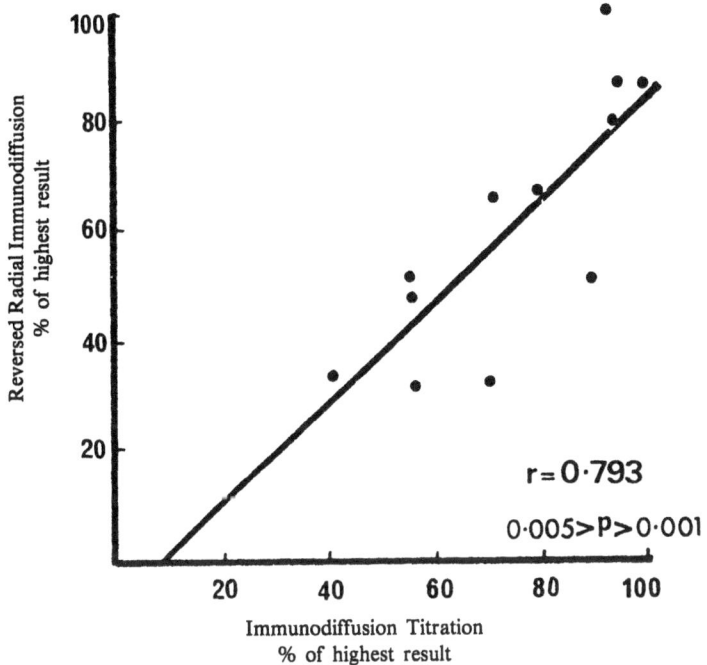

Figure 4.4 Correlation between reversed radial immunodiffusion and immunodiffusion titration testing of sheep anti-human IgG.

Reversed radial immunodiffusion was performed using agar gel containing a standard antigen dilution. Antisera were applied to wells cut in the gel and precipitin ring diameters measured after 18 hours incubation.

Immunodiffusion titration was performed by chequerboard immunodiffusion between a standard antigen solution and antisera, each at twofold reciprocal dilutions between 1 and 32 (i.e. 36 tests per antiserum sample). Precipitin reactions were scored on a scale of 1 to 5 and the results summed to give the antibody content in immunodiffusion titration units.

Laser nephelometry was performed by mixing antisera with successive dilutions of a standard antigen solution in buffer containing polyethylene glycol 6000 (4%) and Tween 20 (0.15%). Results were calculated as the concentration of antigen producing equivalence

significant correlation was obtained between the results of reversed radial immunodiffusion and immunodiffusion titration, which are closely related agar gel techniques. However, no correlation was observed between the results of either of these techniques and those obtained by laser nephelometry (e.g. Figure 4.5).

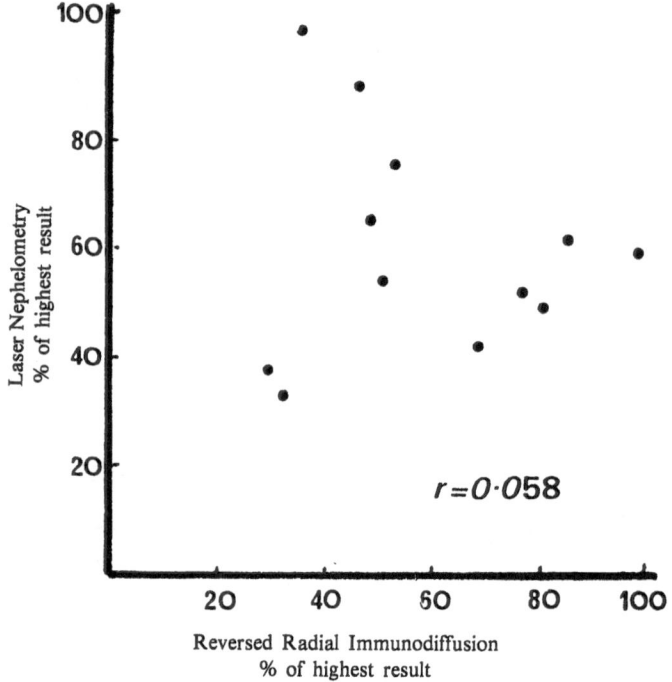

Figure 4.5 Correlation between laser nephelometry and reversed radial immuno-diffusion testing of sheep anti-human IgG. (See Figure 4.4 for key to method)

These results are typical, albeit extreme, of what we have observed in the course of evaluating antisera by immunochemical techniques. Our experiences are by no means unique. Similar results have been reported[10] concerning the suitability of various specific antisera for automated nephelometric procedures. The special characteristics which appear to be required in antibodies for nephelometric applications are not completely understood at present. They may well involve a complex combination of avidity, antibody class and sub-class, the nature of the molecular network formed by the antigen–antibody complexes, and the environment of the test itself.

Even greater differences may be seen when antisera are evaluated by dissimilar techniques. In a study of the involvement of complement in anti-globulin sera[11], little or no correlation was observed between the anti-C3d precipitating and agglutinating activities produced by twelve immunized rabbits. In one extreme case, a rabbit produced a strong agglutinating response despite the absence of detectable precipitating antibodies. Both agglutinating and precipitating activities were associated entirely with the IgG fractions of the rabbit antisera and the observed differences were thought to reflect the intrinsic properties of the antibodies themselves.

4.6 PROCESSING

4.6.1 Absorption

The final stages of antiserum production involve the preparation of pools of suitable antisera for absorption and further processing. As discussed earlier, it is not essential to absorb all antisera as this depends on the types of tests in which they will ultimately be used. However, for most immunochemical applications, absorption is essential. Some years ago it was common practice to carry out this step by adding soluble proteins to precipitate unwanted antibodies. This technique is undesirable because of the possibility of soluble antigen/antibody complexes of residual absorbant, which cannot be removed, causing interaction between antisera[1]. Studies of commercially available anti-IgG, IgA and IgM sera, carried out some years ago[7,8], indicated a substantial number to have been absorbed in this fashion. In recent years, numerous solid-phase absorption techniques have been developed which overcome these disadvantages and antisera intended for routine use should be purified by these methods.

Unfortunately, absorption does not always follow a classical textbook pattern, where the addition of sufficient amounts of insolubilized absorbant removes unwanted antibodies leaving behind only the desired specificity. This is particularly evident with antisera against the four sub-classes of human IgG, where absorption, even under rigorous control of conditions, can easily remove both the unwanted and desired specificities. This is undoubtedly one of the major factors in the absence of availability of these antisera.

4.6.2 Fractionation

Some manufacturers prepare the IgG fraction of the animal antisera, which contains most of the antibody activity. Such fractions offer advantages by virtue of their lower protein concentrations, e.g. in techniques which involve the staining of antiserum-containing gels, where a lower background stain will be obtained. Figure 4.6 shows the results of the electrophoretic separation of six commercially available anti-immunoglobulin sera, prepared in goats, rabbits and sheep. Specimens A and D have been fractionated to varying

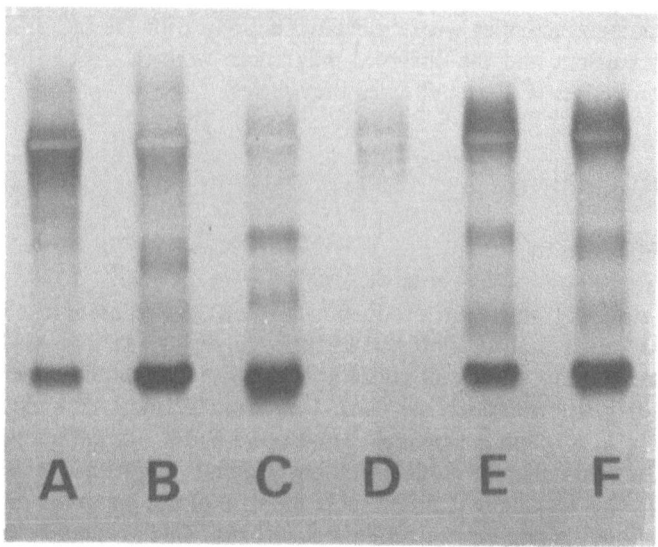

Figure 4.6 Electrophoresis of anti-immunoglobulin sera. Samples A to F represent
six manufacturers' specific anti-immunoglobulin sera. Note the partial fractionation
of sample A, and the extensive fractionation of sample D

extents, but the merits of this processing must be counterbalanced by the
resulting increase in processing costs. Ideally, fractionated antisera should
provide better reagents, but the advantages of such processing can only be
ascertained by reference to the improvements gained, if any, in assay performance.

4.6.3   Additives and presentation

Three general types of additives are found in the processing of antisera.
Firstly, antimicrobial agents such as azide or merthiolate, secondly, residues
of reagents used in delipidization and fractionation processes, and thirdly,
agents which stabilize the antisera or enhance their reactivity with their
corresponding antigens. A good example of the latter is found with many
antiglobulin reagents used in semi-automatic spin-Coombs techniques.
Figure 4.7 shows the electrophoretic separation of two such antisera, prepared
in rabbits, compared with an untreated rabbit antiglobulin serum. The patterns
of these two antisera, which are typical of several available commercially,
reveal that the antisera have been fractionated, diluted and contain substantial

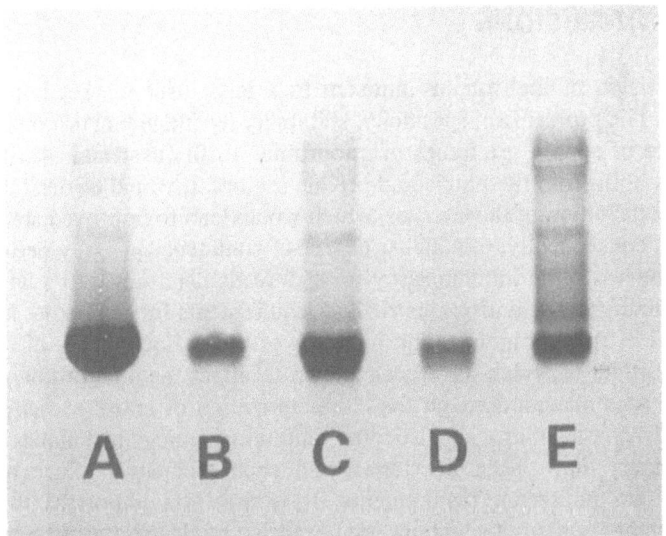

Figure 4.7 Electrophoresis of antiglobulin (Coombs) sera. Samples A to D represent two manufacturers' antiglobulin (Coombs) sera:
A = manufacturer 1, concentrated × 20
B = manufacturer 1, not concentrated
C = manufacturer 2, concentrated × 10
D = manufacturer 2, not concentrated
E = untreated antiglobulin serum

amounts of an albumin additive. This albumin can be shown by immuno-electrophoresis to be of bovine origin. While such antisera may be acceptable for semi-automated antiglobulin techniques it would be unwise to use them in other antiglobulin techniques or immunochemical methods without a strict evaluation of their suitability.

The final stage of antiserum production is the presentation, which can eventually take the form of frozen, freeze-dried or liquid material. While the liquid form is most convenient to use it has a shorter storage life and due care must be given to this point. Frozen antisera are less convenient to use and are subject to the vagaries of low temperature storage, but freeze-dried antisera are likely to have the longest storage life, prior to reconstitution. A most important feature of antiserum storage, and one frequently neglected, is the avoidance of repeated freezing and thawing. Antisera should be stored frozen in order to avoid denaturation effects.

4.7   CONCLUSIONS

The provision of high quality antisera to a large user market is a complex exercise. The problems of specificity, suitability for individual test methods and guarantee of supply are issues of importance to the user and also to manufacturers both from the public and private sectors. It would be desirable to see a greater definition of these issues, which would lead to improved standardization and, consequently, to a higher degree of confidence in assay performance.

The success of all immunoassay procedures is determined to a large extent by the quality of the antisera used. The requirements for antibodies have been discussed in this communication in terms of the various stages of antiserum production, all of which have been shown to affect the final product. Since a series of recommendations on the characterization of antisera was published in 1971[1], newer, more sophisticated immunochemical techniques such as nephelometry have been developed and such techniques place additional demands on antiserum requirements. It is therefore important that future developments in assay techniques are paralleled by developments in antiserum production, and a greater insight into those features which determine the suitability of antisera for individual methods.

Acknowledgements

I acknowledge and appreciate the contributions made by Margaret J. C. Fergusson, Robin H. Fraser, Joe W. McCallum and J. Graham Templeton to the work reported herein, and for assistance in preparing the manuscript.

References

1. MRC Working Party (1971). Recommendations made on the clinical use of immunological reagents. *Immunology*, **20**, 3
2. Fergusson, M., Hunter, I., Munro, A. C. and Watt, A. (1977). Problems associated with the production of anti-immunoglobulin sera. Presented at *Scotblood '77*, February 26, Edinburgh
3. Powell, L. W., Alpert, E., Isselbacher, K. J. and Drysdale, J. W. (1975). Human isoferritins: organ specific iron and apoferritin distribution. *Br. J. Haematol.*, **30**, 47
4. Hazard, J. T., Yokota, M., Arosio, P. and Drysdale, J. W. (1977). Immunologic differences in human isoferritins: complications for immunologic quantitation of serum ferritin. *Blood*, **49**, 139
5. Van der Giessen, M., de Lange, B. and Van der Lee, B. (1974). The production of precipitating antiglobulin reagents specific for the sub-classes of human IgG. *Immunology*, **27**, 655

6. Beck, M. L. and Marsh, W. L. (1977). Complement and the antiglobulin. *Transfusion*, **17**, 529

7. Reimer, C. B., Phillips, D. J., Maddison, S. E. and Shore, S. L. (1970). Comparative evaluation of commercial precipitating antisera against human IgM and IgG. *J. Lab. Clin. Med.*, **76**, 949

8. Phillips, D. J., Shore, S. L., Maddison, S. E., Gordon, D. S. and Reimer, C. B. (1971). Comparative evaluation of commercial precipitating antisera against human IgA. *J. Lab. Clin. Med.*, **77**, 639

9. Reimer, C. B. and Maddison, S. E. (1976). Standardization of human immunoglobulin quantitation: a review of current status and problems. *Clin. Chem.*, **22**, 577

10. Ritchie, R. F. (1972). Evaluation of antibody preparations for the AIP system. Presented at the *Colloquium on AIP*, May 2, Brussels

11. Moore, J. A. and Chaplin, H. Jr. (1974). Anti-C3d antiglobulin reagents I. Characteristics of the anti-C3c and anti-C3d responses during hyperimmunization in rabbits. *Transfusion*, **14**, 407

5

Problems encountered in immunochemical technique methodology
J. T. Whicher

5.1 INTRODUCTION   52

5.2 ACCURACY   52
    5.2.1 *Antigen fragments: C3 assay*   53
    5.2.2 *Antigenic mixtures: paraprotein assay*   54
    5.2.3 *Allotypes: haptoglobin assay*   56

5.3 PRECISION   57

5.4 SENSITIVITY   58

5.5 ANTISERUM REQUIREMENTS   58

5.6 ANALYTE REQUIREMENTS   59

5.7 SPEED   59

5.8 SUMMARY   60

5.1 INTRODUCTION

Immunochemical methods are capable of a high degree of sensitivity and specificity. Such methods are, however, influenced by the nature of both the antibody and antigen.

For ideal performance, immunochemical measuring systems require mono-specific antisera, a single homogeneous test protein and standards which behave in an identical fashion to the test in the assay system. In fact, these criteria are rarely all met[1], and give rise to a number of practical problems.

5.2 ACCURACY

Accuracy in immunochemical systems is dependent upon the molecular characteristics of the antigen, the specificity of the antiserum and the physical principle of the method (Table 5.1). For these reasons it is fruitless to discuss the accuracy of such methods without reference to the analyte in question. The antiserum used in an assay may be specific for a certain protein but, because sera contain varying amounts of physically different molecules (e.g. polymers or fragments), methods dependent on different molecular charac-teristics (e.g. nephelometry or Laurell rockets) will give different answers when the same standard is used. A large part of the problem can be put down

TABLE 5.1 Factors affecting the accuracy of immunochemical methods

Nature	Examples
Analyte	
antigenic mixtures	immunoglobulins
substance bound to antigen	lipoprotein B/lipid
antigen polymers/aggregates	IgM
antigen fragments	C3, C4
allotypes	haptoglobin
Assay	
antibody variation	titre, affinity, specificity
gel techniques	effects of molecular size
electrophoretic techniques	charge effects
Standard	
difficulty in assigning weight values	difference between standards
molecular heterogeneity	dissimilar behaviour to test sample

to the fact that the standard and test material are not identical and thus show dissimilar comparative behaviour in different assays. Some of the factors contributing to these effects are shown in Table 5.1. They will be illustrated by the use of some commonly encountered examples.

5.2.1 Antigen fragments: C3 assay

The C3 molecule has a number of antigens (Figure 5.1). Activation either by physiological complement conversion or breakdown *in vitro* by proteolytic

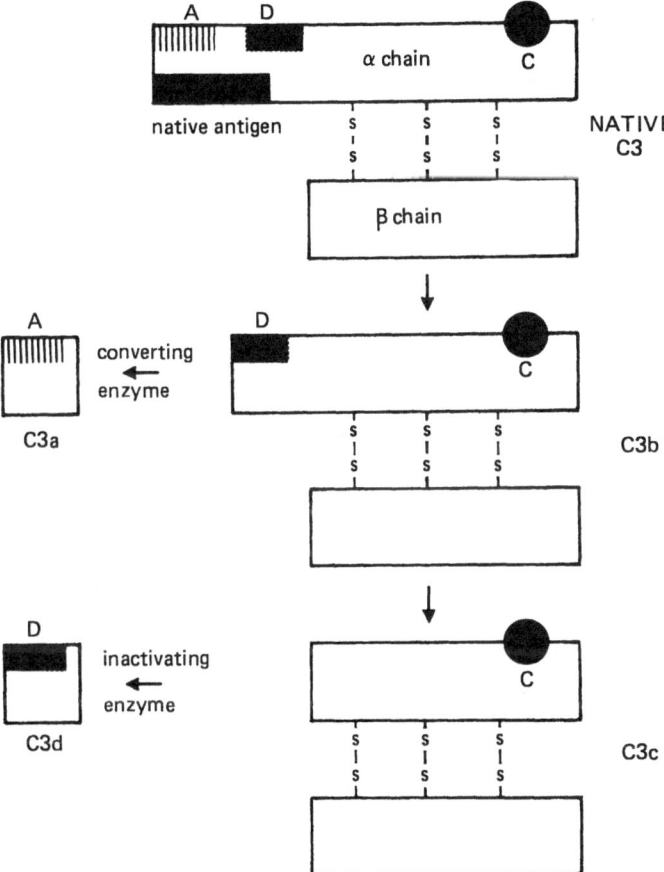

Figure 5.1 Antigenic changes during activation and inactivation of C3. Four antigens are present: A, C, D and native. These are segregated onto different-sized fragments during cleavage of the molecule

enzymes such as plasmin result in segregation of antigens onto different sized fragments of C3. The fragments possess differing charge, antigenic reactivity and molecular size from the native molecules and their presence gives rise to inaccuracy in C3 assay by some methods. For example, when fresh serum was compared with serum 'aged' for 3 days at 37 °C, the aged serum gave a value 50% higher than the fresh serum when assayed for C3 by radial immuno-diffusion[2]. Similar but less marked changes will occur during storage of samples at room temperature (for example during transit to the laboratory). These effects are probably due to the fact that the conversion products of C3, C3c and C3d are of lower molecular weight than native C3 and diffuse into the gel more rapidly. When the same comparison was made by Laurell rockets, a 10% difference was seen. In this case molecular size is unimportant and the difference is probably due to the higher negative charge on C3c and to the availability of different antigenic determinants consuming more anti-bodies[3]. Clearly the presence of conversion products *in vivo* or *in vitro* may cause an overestimation of C3 in exactly the situation where low levels are being sought.

The measurement of C3 thus provides a good example of a number of analyte factors and how they interact with two assay types. It is interesting to note that free fluid-phase nephelometric techniques do not appear to be affected by these problems.

5.2.2 Antigenic mixtures: paraprotein assay

It is important to assay paraproteins for the follow-up of patients and to assess the probability of malignancy[4]. Immunochemical techniques give very variable results between methods and consistent results for a single method may only be obtained if a single batch of antiserum is used. Antisera to immunoglobulins are largely directed against the determinants in the Fc region of the molecules[5]. Paraproteins are only of a single immunoglobulin subtype and G_m type and frequently show deletions which render their C_H domains antigenically different from their polyclonal counterparts[6]. This results in the selective consumption of the antibody population of an anti-immunoglobulin antiserum which in the Laurell rocket and radial immunodiffusion assays may cause gross overestimates of paraprotein concentration, sometimes greater than serum total protein. Monoclonal antigens frequently show non-parallel dilution curves (Figure 5.2). In the immunodiffusion technique the ring of diffusion may rapidly pass across the whole plate selectively depleting it of antibody and possibly giving rise to inaccuracy in other samples on the same plate. An important problem is the fact that, in some nephelometric systems, an unsuspected paraprotein may pass into antigen excess (Figure 5.2) and give any result, depending on its position on the precipitin curve. The only reasonable solution to these problems is to electrophorese all samples which may contain paraproteins. The methods for antigen excess detection in nephelo-

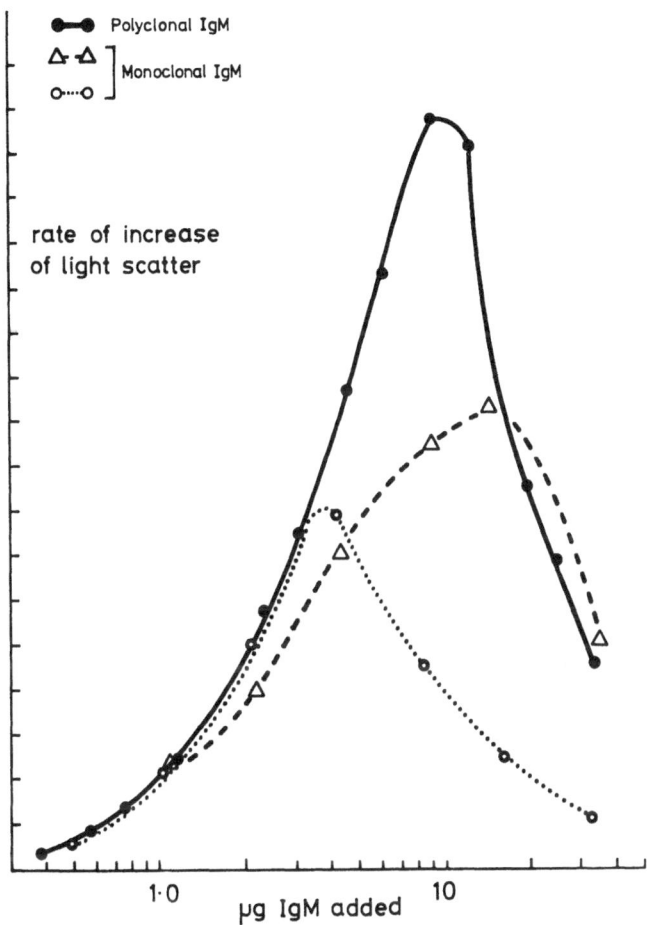

Figure 5.2   Dilution curve of two IgM paraproteins in a rate nephelometric system compared with that of a polyclonal standard. Paraprotein concentrations are calculated from the most dilute aliquot which can be read with confidence from the standard curve. Both paraproteins pass into antigen excess at lower levels of estimated IgM protein than the polyclonal standard suggesting selective consumption of antibody. It can be seen that paraprotein A shows a dilution curve that is not parallel to the other materials

metric systems, while reliable, are time consuming and best avoided[7,8]. They depend on the addition of further antigen or antibody in order to ascertain whether there is free antibody remaining within the system. The technique used in a rate reaction system[9] is shown in Figure 5.3. Paraproteins are thus examples of a situation in which a mixture of antigens is being measured, and when only a single component of the mixture predominates the measurement becomes inaccurate.

5.2.3   Allotypes: haptoglobin assay

Haptoglobin is composed of four polypeptide chains: two α chains and two β chains. A large number of allotypes have been described which fall into three families designated Hp1-1, Hp2-1 and Hp2-2, depending on the general

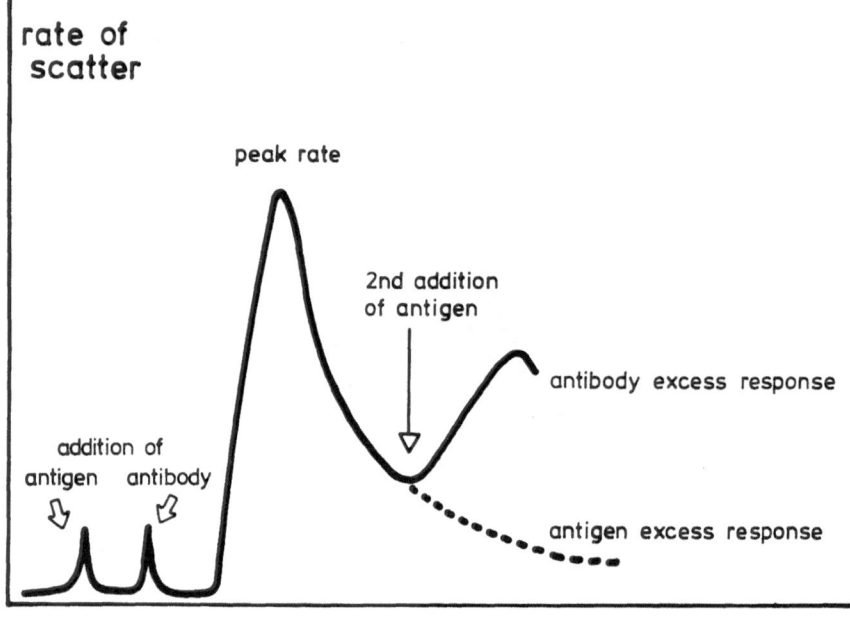

Figure 5.3   Method of testing for antigen excess in a rate of reaction nephelometric system[8]. Antigen and antibody are added to the cuvette and a peak rate of increase of light scattering is developed. This falls off to leave a constant amount of light scattering. If further antigen is now added a new rate will be seen if residual antibody is present; if however the initial was in antigen excess there will be no subsequent rate

structure of the alpha chains. Hp1-1 is a monomer but Hp2-1 and Hp2-2 show a series of polymeric forms. The European population shows a preponderance of the Hp^2 gene, whereas Nigerians show a high incidence of the Hp^1 gene, Immunochemical measurement is thus faced with the problem of genetic variants, all of which occur commonly in the population. They have different antigenic determinants and different molecular sizes. Gel techniques tend to underestimate the polymeric allotypes Hp2-1 and Hp2-2 in comparison with Hp1-1. The Laurell rocket technique gives values 20% too low for Hp2-2. The errors in the radial immunodiffusion technique decrease with incubation time as more complete diffusion can occur. There is virtually no difference between the phenotypes using nephelometric techniques.

These examples have been used to show some of the problems encountered in the immunochemical measurement of plasma proteins. Many problems are due to the *molecular heterogeneity* either in a single test sample or in a population of test samples. The heterogeneity may be genetic, generated by a disease process or created *in vitro* after the specimen has been taken from the patient.

5.3 PRECISION

Poor precision is a problem in *routine* immunochemical systems and reflects the large number of manual procedures that are involved. Most laboratories would find a between-batch coefficient of variation of 10–15% for the radial immunodiffusion technique, while the Laurell rocket technique, with more easily measured peaks, gives a coefficient of variation of 5–10%. Nephelo-metric systems are, not surprisingly, better with a coefficient of variation of 5% and show far more consistent results between laboratories, particularly if they are automated. Imprecision is a summation of the errors involved in every step in the analytical system; for example the precision of the RID technique depends on

(a) the initial sample dilution
(b) the filling of the well with a small volume of analyte
(c) the reading of the precipitation ring
(d) plotting and reading of the samples from the standard curve.

In general, the two major features which may improve precision are the use of automatic diluters and a computed curve fit and test value calculation. It is therefore unreasonable to discuss the precision of different immunochemical assay systems as though it were inherent in the method, because it is often due to ancillary routines such as those mentioned. For example, it is well known that the precision of the RID system is improved by longer incubation;

this is due to improved visibility of precipitin rings and to the fact that the standard curve becomes steeper, improving the manual reading of test samples from it. It is possible to achieve a between-batch CV of about 2%.

5.4 SENSITIVITY

Sensitivity in most immunochemical systems is largely dependent upon antibody titre and affinity and the ability to detect small amounts of antigen/antibody precipitate without interference.

Radial immunodiffusion and Laurell rocket techniques, with conventional staining, will detect as little as $0.5–0.1\,\mu$g of antigen applied to the plate when using high affinity antibodies (approximately 1 mg/l of antigen in plasma). Neat plasma can usually be used in gel systems. If radio-labelled antibodies are used, the detection limit goes down to $0.05–0.01\,\mu$g of antigen (0.1 mg/l of antigen in plasma).

Nephelometric techniques are limited in their sensitivity by background-light scattering particles in plasma generating a low signal-to-noise ratio. It is thus usually impossible to use neat plasma or serum even if it is filtered, but neat urine or CSF may be used. For example, in urine the Hyland PDQ nephelometer will comfortably measure 0.1 mg/l of IgG. Rate reaction systems may overcome the problem of background light scattering to a greater extent.

5.5 ANTISERUM REQUIREMENTS

Antiserum for radial immunodiffusion may be of a relatively poor titre and affinity for a workable method to be achieved. Specificity is more important as it may be difficult to visualize multiple rings. However, trace contaminants do not usually present a problem.

Antiserum requirements are not rigorous for the Laurell rocket technique. Poor specificity results in multiple peaks which can easily be recognized and ignored. In fact bispecific antisera may be used to measure two proteins simultaneously. High titre and affinity gives clearer peaks and better sensitivity but crude antisera are quite usable.

Available systems for nephelometry either measure light scattering after a period of time, usually when the amount of scatter is static, or measure the rate of increase of scattering. Antiserum must be of high affinity to work well in all these systems, though the use of polyethylene glycol enhances antibody–antigen interaction. Monospecificity is extremely important, as any contaminating antibodies will form complexes with their respective antigens and will be included in the final measured value[10].

5.6 ANALYTE REQUIREMENTS

(a) *Radial immunodiffusion*—Antigens containing varying amounts of polymer will suffer severe inaccuracy, e.g. 19S IgM gives only 30% of the assay value of the same amount of 7S protein[1]. Paraproteins present a problem in that they may give no ring of precipitation owing to the migration of soluble antibody–antigen complexes to the edge of the plate. This may deplete the plate of antiserum.

(b) *Laurell rockets*—Antigens with molecular weights of less than 50 000 are generally less suitable for this technique as they rapidly diffuse during electrophoresis, giving rise to very wide rockets which may fuse with each other[1]. Molecular charge and size heterogeneity will both affect this method slightly but problems are not usually severe. Antigens with anodal mobility at pH 8.6 (e.g. immunoglobulins) require alteration by formylation or carbamylation prior to assay[1,9]: The support medium may also be modified[11]. Paraproteins pass off the top of the plate and are usually easily recognized.

(c) *Nephelometry*—The molecular characteristics of the antigen seem to be of less importance in nephelometric assays than in gel techniques. Antigen excess does not cause major problems in gel techniques as it results in the precipitate being driven off the plate, a situation which is easily recognizable. In nephelometric techniques, antigen excess may give rise to any value depending on where on the precipitin curve the sample falls. It is probable that the only antigens which will consume all the available antibodies are paraproteins and thus it is only in immunoglobulin measurement that this is likely to be a problem. Continuous flow systems usually show characteristic peak profiles in antigen excess[12].

Light-scattering particles such as lipoproteins provide background scatter which limits the sensitivity of nephelometric systems for the measurement of proteins in plasma. It also may give rise to the need to measure blank values on sera which are not at high dilution.

5.7 SPEED

(a) *Radial immunodiffusion*—Speed of assays is slow with a minimum diffusion time of 16 hours. Diffusion rate may, however, be increased by incubation at 37°C.

(b) *Laurell rocket*—Assays may be performed in as little as two hours for proteins with high anodal mobilities, e.g. albumin. Six hours is more usual but 16 hours does not require cooling and gives better precipitation (by allowing longer for antibody–antigen interaction to occur).

(c) *Nephelometric techniques*—These may be very quick and some are easily automated, thus giving large throughput and improved precision.

5.8 SUMMARY

The problems of immunochemical techniques are due largely to the inherent molecular heterogeneity of most plasma proteins. This gives rise to heterogeneity in antisera raised against these proteins and in reference material derived from them. The result of these factors depends upon the interaction with the physical principle of the assay system. The immunochemical assay systems have enormous versatility if these factors are appreciated and taken account of.

References

1. Laurell, C. B. (1972). Electroimmunoassay. *Scand. J. Clin. Lab. Invest.*, **29**, suppl. 124, 21
2. Alper, C. A. and Rosen, F. S. (1975). Clinical applications of complement assays. *Adv. Intern. Med.*, **20**, 61
3. Vladutiu, A. O. (1975). C3 standards. *Lancet*, **i**, 979
4. Hobbs, J. R. (1971). Immunoglobulins in clinical chemistry. *Adv. Clin. Chem.*, **14**, 219
5. Grubb, A. (1973). Immunochemical quantitation of IgG: Influences of the antiserum and of the antigenic population. *Scand. J. Clin. Lab. Invest.*, **31**, 465
6. Porter, R. R. (1969). Structure of immunoglobulin heavy chain. In Franck, F. and Shugar, D. (ed.). *Gammaglobulins. Structure and Biosynthesis*, p. 13–19. (London and New York: Academic Press)
7. Deaton, C. D., Maxwell, K. W., Smith, R. S. and Creveling, R. L. (1973). Use of laser nephelometry in the measurements of serum proteins. *Clin. Chem.*, **22**, 1465
8. Sternberg, J. C. (1977). A rate nephelometer for measuring specific proteins by immunoprecipitans reaction. *Clin. Chem.*, **23**, No. 8 1456
9. Slater, L. (1975). IgG, IgA and IgM by formylated rocket immunoelectrophoresis. *Ann. Clin. Biochem.*, **12**, 19
10. Weeke, B. (1968). Carbamylated human immunoglobulins tested by electrophoresis in agarose and antibody–containing agarose. *Scand. J. Clin. Lab. Invest.*, **21**, 351

11. Schuller, E., Lefevre, M. and Tömpe, L. (1972). Electroimmunodiffusion of α_2M, IgA and IgM in nanogram quantities with a hydroxyethyl cellulose–agarose gel: Applications to unconcentrated C.S.F. *Clin. Chim. Acta*, **42**, 5
12. Ritchie, R. F. (1975). Automated immunoprecipitation analysis of serum proteins. In Putnam, F. W. (ed.). *The Plasma Proteins*. (New York: Academic Press)

6

Specific protein measurement and standardization

R. S. Wainwright, J. R. Doggart and
D. W. Neill

6.1   INTRODUCTION   64

6.2   NEED FOR STANDARDIZATION IN PROTEIN
      ASSAYS   64

6.3   STANDARDIZATION AS A CONCEPT   70

6.4   ACCEPTANCE OF STANDARDIZATION   70

6.5   THE COLLABORATIVE APPROACH TO
      STANDARDIZATION   71

6.6   DISADVANTAGES AND ADVANTAGES OF
      STANDARDIZATION   72

6.7   STANDARDIZATION OF NEW TECHNIQUES   72

6.1   INTRODUCTION

For much of the argument presented in this paper we are indebted to a variety of sources. Many of the points have already been made in correspondence in the News Sheet of the Association of Clinical Biochemists; one result of this correspondence has been the setting up of an Analytical Methods Working Party.

6.2   NEED FOR STANDARDIZATION IN PROTEIN ASSAYS

The need for standardization is evident from the results of inter-laboratory surveys and quality control schemes (Figures 6.1 to 6.5). Belk and Sunderman[1] described the variation of results obtained when prepared albumin and total protein standard (4.6 g/100 ml and 6.6 g/100 ml respectively) were estimated in 59 laboratories during a survey of accuracy of chemical analyses in clinical laboratories in the state of Pennsylvania. The range of values recorded for albumin was from 1.5 to 10 g/100 ml and for total protein from 4.5 to 12 g/ 100 ml.

Figure 6.1a and Figure 6.1b are recent examples taken from the National Quality Control Scheme for albumin and total protein. Histogram distributions with unit increments (g/l) between 23–33 for albumin and 57–71 for total protein are presented against the number of laboratories reporting given values. The histograms take no account of the methods of estimation. More detailed data are also provided, with inclusion of mean, standard deviation and coefficient of variation for each of the most commonly used methods. Clearly in each case the range of results is unacceptably wide. Further, grossly differing mean values with coefficients of variation approaching 10% for individual methods cast serious doubt on the accuracy and validity of routine procedures.

Figure 6.2a and Figure 6.2b are examples taken from the Wellcome Quality Control Scheme, again for albumin and total protein. They provide similar evidence to Figure 6.1a and Figure 6.1b above. No account is taken of individual methodologies. Albumin, determined by a variety of methods in 792 laboratories had a value of $32.8 \pm 3.5(SD)$ g/l. Eleven laboratories within this group, using a particular method (BCG on the Technicon SMAC Analyser showed a mean of $38.8 \pm 4.7(SD)$ g/l). The corresponding result for total protein determined by a variety of methods in 909 laboratories was 64.5 ± 3.0 (SD) g/l whereas for 201 laboratories using a Biuret procedure the values were $66.0 \pm 2.1(SD)$ g/l.

NATIONAL QUALITY CONTROL SCHEME
(ALBUMIN)

HISTOGRAM DISTRIBUTION FOR ALBUMIN

```
| •••• | •••• | •••• | •••• | •••• | •••• | •••• |
*                                        *
*                              • • • • • •    MINIMUM VALUE        10
*                         XXXX*              23                    6
*                          XXX*              24                    6
*                       XXXXXXX*             25                   14
*            XXXXXXXXXXXXXXXXXXXXXXX*         26                   34
*    XXXXXXXXXXXXXXXXXXXXXXXXXXXXXXX*         27                   62
*           XXXXXXXXXXXXXXXXXXXXXXX*          28                   48
*          XXXXXXXXXXXXXXXXXXXXXXX*           29                   53
*              XXXXXXXXXXXXXX*                30                   29
*                        XXXXX*              31                   11
*                          XXX*              32                    6
*                             *              33                    1
*                      • • • • • •   MAXIMUM VALUE                 8
*                                        *
*                                        *
| •••• | •••• | •••• | •••• | •••• | •••• | •••• |
70    60    50    40    30    20    10    NUMBER OF RESULTS
NUMBER OF RESULTS IN HISTOGRAM     288
```

RESULTS FOR ALBUMIN (g/l)
(EXCLUDING VALUES OUTSIDE 3 SD FOR METHOD)

METHOD	NO. OF VALUES	MEAN	STD. DEV.	C. OF VAR.
ELECTROPHORESIS SCANNING	8	27.6	2.8	10.2
MANUAL − B.C.G.	63	27.8	2.7	9.8
OTHER	30	26.6	5.0	18.6
AUTOANALYSER I−BCG	53	27.9	1.8	6.6
AA II OR SMA SYSTEM−BCG	105	27.8	1.9	6.9
VICKERS M300 D300	23	27.5	1.1	4.1

Figure 6.1a Example of National Quality Control Scheme for albumin presented as a histogram distribution and as a series of results sub-divided into different methods of estimation

From these data it is clear that different methods are accompanied by different bias, and that gross imprecision and inaccuracy may invalidate established procedures.

Figure 6.3 provides an example of the West of Scotland Immunoglobulin Control Programme. Two sera, A and B, each containing immunoglobulins IgG, IgA and IgM were analysed by a series of laboratories denoted by numbers 2–35 and letters A–G. Means, standard deviations, and coefficients of variation illustrate the gross imprecision of measurement of specific proteins.

NATIONAL QUALITY CONTROL SCHEME
(TOTAL PROTEIN)

HISTOGRAM DISTRIBUTION FOR TOTAL PROTEIN

```
|****|****|****|****|****|****|****|
-
*                           *
*                           *
*                           *
*                    . . .*      MINIMUM VALUE        9
*                     XX*           57                8
*                   XXXXX*          59                16
*               XXXXXXXXXXX*        61                35
*    XXXXXXXXXXXXXXXXXXXXXXXXXXXXX* 63                82
*        XXXXXXXXXXXXXXXXXXXXXXXXX* 65                69
*         XXXXXXXXXXXXXXXXXXXXXXX*  67                64
*                   XXXXXX*         69                19
*                      XX*          71                6
*                         *      MAXIMUM VALUE        5
*                         *
*                         *
*                         *

|****|****|****|****|****|****|****|
105    90    75    60    45    30    15      NUMBER OF RESULTS
   NUMBER OF RESULTS IN HISTOGRAM   313
```

RESULTS FOR TOTAL PROTEIN (g/l)
(EXCLUDING VALUES OUTSIDE 3 SD FOR METHOD)

METHOD	NO. OF VALUES	MEAN	STD. DEV.	C.OF VAR.
MANUAL BIURET	81	62.5	3.3	5.3
REFRACTOMETER	7	58.6	2.4	3.5
OTHER	19	60.9	4.5	7.3
AUTOANALYSER I BIURET	60	66.0	2.6	4.0
AA II OR SMA BIURET	120	65.7	2.6	3.9
VICKERS M300 D300	23	63.3	2.0	3.2

Figure 6.1b Example of National Quality Control Scheme for total protein presented as a histogram distribution and as a series of results sub-divided into different methods of estimation

Figure 6.4 and Figure 6.5 demonstrate similar findings related to α-feto-protein. Figure 6.4 taken from the AFP Quality Control Scheme compares α-fetoprotein results obtained in 26 laboratories with those obtained in 8 'reference' laboratories denoted as such by virtue of their lower imprecision in earlier surveys. All results are compared with expected or 'target' values.

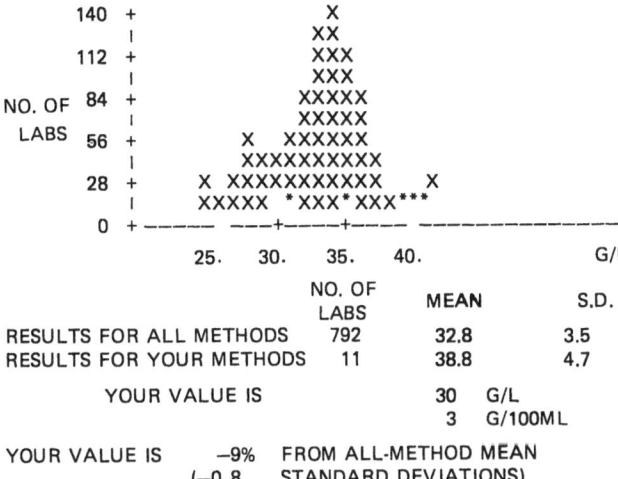

Figure 6.2a Example of Wellcome Quality Control Scheme for albumin presented as a histogram distribution. Statistics are calculated (a) for all methods (b) for the method employed in the particular laboratory included (BCG)

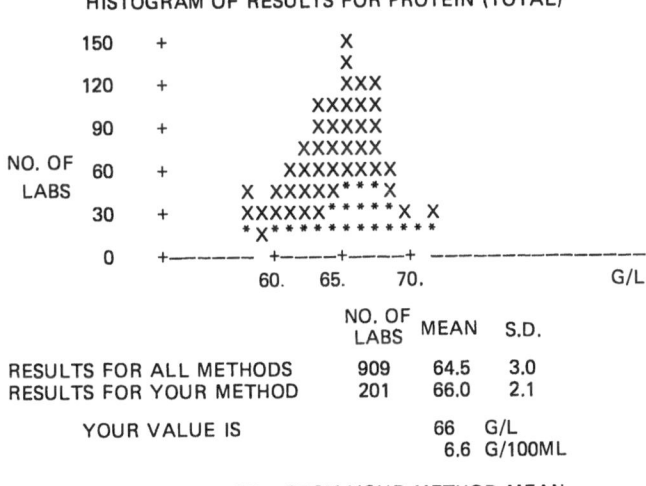

Figure 6.2b Example of Wellcome Quality Control Scheme for total protein presented as a histogram distribution. Statistics are calculated (a) for all methods (b) for the method employed in the particular laboratory included (Biuret)

		B	C	D	E	G
A	IgG	6.45	11.9	8.20	7.40	6.2
	IgA	0.63	0.82	1.02	1.00	0.6
	IgM	0.92	0.80	0.84	0.54	0.8
B	IgG	6.70	11.31	7.40	10.3	6.5
	IgA	0.67	0.87	0.96	1.14	0.6
	IgM	11.10	5.91	8.80	9.5	8.0

		2	4	5	8	14	17	18	19	25	35	A
A	IgG	8.28	6.1	7.6	7.84	7.5	7.2	8.51	5.50	8.72	6.6	5.4
	IgA	0.40	0.61	0.8	0.83	1.1	0.82	0.91	0.90	0.86	0.7	0.7
	IgM	0.32	0.82	0.8	0.85	0.7	0.96	1.05	0.55	0.94	0.8	0.8
B	IgG	8.16	6.1	7.7	7.84	7.2	7.2	10.5	5.0	7.44	6.1	5.8
	IgA	0.70	0.61	0.8	0.88	0.9	0.82	0.79	0.80	0.74	0.7	0.5
	IgM	7.20	8.1	9.7	9.82	7.8	9.8	7.76	3.0	1.84	8.4	3.35

		Mean	SD	CV
A	IgG	7.463	1.574	21.1
	IgA	0.794	0.181	22.8
	IgM	0.781	0.181	23.2
B	IgG	7.578	3.116	41.1
	IgA	0.780	0.156	20.0
	IgM	8.231	1.923	23.4

Figure 6.3 An example of the West of Scotland Immunoglobulin Control Programme. Individual results and calculated statistics for two sera A and B containing immunoglobulins IgG, IgA and IgM distributed to a variety of laboratories are presented. The individual laboratories are labelled 2–35 and A–G

Target Value (U/l)		50	75	100	125
Total Group (N 26)					
Mean	(U/l)	52.1	73.4	102	122
SD	(U/l)	9.0	14.7	20.6	27.2
CV	(%)	17.3	20.0	20.2	22.3
'Reference' Group (N 8)*					
Mean	(U/l)	50.4	70.0	103	123
SD	(U/l)	6.7	8.2	14.6	23.1
CV	(%)	13.3	11.7	14.2	18.9

Figure 6.4   Example of AFP quality control scheme (Edinburgh)

*The 'Reference Group' is composed of a series of laboratories (N = 8) who had achieved greatest precision during an earlier stage of the scheme.

Laboratory	(stated value, µg/l)	Lab A	Lab B	Lab C	Lab D
A	(200)	222	230	193	127
B	(160)	217	210	114	106
C	(110)	100	65	73	109
D	(160)	275	190	228	149

Figure 6.5   Accuracy of AFP results on standards from four laboratories

Figure 6.5 compares the accuracy of estimation of four α-fetoprotein 'standards' A, B, C and D taken from four laboratories A, B, C and D and recirculated so that each laboratory would estimate all four standards.

Again, serious discrepancies are obvious; e.g. standard B assayed in laboratory A gave a result more than twice that of laboratory D. Similar findings occurred when standard D was assayed in laboratories A and D whereas laboratory D provided higher values than laboratory A for standard C.

We can only reiterate what Watson and Pow[2] have said in relation to AFP: 'Clearly, the assay is a shambles. The need for more extensive quality control of diagnostic reagents sets would seem to be obvious'. And one can extend these criticisms to all protein assays and to other reagents in addition to those supplied in kit form.

Further, standardization is being demanded by 'the consumer'. Thus G. R. Cooper, of the National Communicable Disease Center of the US Department of Health, Education and Welfare, said in 1968[3] that 'clinical disciplines are taking considerable interest in laboratory standardization. International clinical groups interested in cardiovascular diseases, diabetes, mental diseases and other chronic diseases have commented repeatedly on the need for better control and standardization systems in the laboratory to support their clinical and epidemiological investigations'.

With apologies to J. P. Cali[4] of the National Bureau of Standards, Washington, let us imagine a Scotsman in Inverness or Aberdeen who had a medical history built up over a few years, including immunoglobulin results from one specific laboratory. For business reasons he now has to go into exile south of the border where clinical follow-up continues, including immuno-globulin results from another laboratory. Both laboratories may have produced highly precise results on the patient, but unless both laboratories are pro-ducing *accurate* results, no mechanism exists for comparison of their results over time and distance.

Points similar to this have been recognized for decades by analysts outside clinical laboratories, but, what is more, these same analysts have − also for decades − been working purposefully towards the elimination of factors which give rise to discrepancies between laboratories, by the standardization of analytical methods.

6.3   STANDARDIZATION AS A CONCEPT

This leads us to a possible definition of what we mean by the standardization of analytical methods. Could it be, to use the words of H. Egan[5], 'to achieve a uniform method of laboratory procedure as a means of obtaining consistent analytical results between individual workers, and, in particular, individual laboratories'?

That quotation has been taken slightly out of context, but it does, we think, give some idea of what is meant by standardization. Opinions may differ on the extent to which standardization should be applied, but, to quote again, this time from the remarks of the chairman of a symposium on the subject, reported in 1950[6], 'some degree of standardization is implicit in all scientific work and it is, therefore, an essential factor in the advancement and expansion of the practice of chemistry'. We may refer later to the aspect of 'advancement and expansion'.

6.4   ACCEPTANCE OF STANDARDIZATION

Now let us look briefly at areas where the concept of standardization has long been accepted. One area which affects most of us at some time during our lives is that of fine *chemicals,* and, more particularly, those fine chemicals which are destined for medicinal use. 'Standards of purity, of nomenclature and of definition for medicinal substances became necessary for the protection of the public and as a basis of understanding between the physician and the pharmacist who dispensed his prescriptions"[7]. (One may ask, in passing, 'What about the basis of understanding between the physician and the laboratory worker on whose results the physician relies? Or does he?').

The interesting point is that such standards began to be laid down even before 1864, when the first British Pharmacopoeia came into existence. This publication and its companion, the British Pharmaceutical Codex, contain analytical methods which must be used and which can be relied on.

Another class of product is that which comprises *analytical reagents*. We know how often we have to check a label so as to be sure that a reagent is suitable for our purpose, and many of the analytical methods used in ensuring that the reagents meet certain criteria are published in book form by the manufacturers.

Many of us have already to some extent accepted the concept of standardization in our own field almost without knowing it, by accepting and using pituitary hormone standards, whose assigned values have been agreed by international collaboration. Further, the Expert Panel on Proteins of the International Federation of Clinical Chemistry has assigned[8], or hopes to assign, values to a reference serum, 74/1, for α_1-antitrypsin, C3, IgA, IgG, IgE, IgM and transferrin.

6.5 THE COLLABORATIVE APPROACH TO STANDARDIZATION

Use of the word 'collaboration' brings us to our next point, which is that the development of acceptable uniform methods of analysis demands the collaboration of many laboratory workers. Rodgerson and Tietz[9] have stated something which many of us would be forced to agree with—that, in some cases, there has been no evidence presented that a newly selected method has a clinical usefulness equal to, or better than, that which it replaces. 'There is today possibly more confusion than at any time in the past, and this is being exacerbated by the decreasing ability of many laboratories to perform comprehensive evaluation of methods because of the pressures and demands of service work.'

So there has to be collaborative, co-ordinated effort directed by, preferably, professional organizations. The Society of Public Analysts has been working in this way since 1924 at least, although it was thought at first that standardization of analytical methods was impracticable because of the large amount of specialized work entailed; it was certainly seen as a long-term process.

The Institute of Petroleum started similar work in 1920 and produces each year two updated volumes of methods. The Association of Official Analytical Chemists in the USA has long been operating in a similar way. Other professional bodies could be mentioned.

6.6 DISADVANTAGES AND ADVANTAGES OF STANDARDIZATION

(a) Standardized methods may be too cumbersome for routine use.

This criticism need not carry any weight if we can distinguish between reference methods and routine methods. The reference methods are 'highly defined rigid procedures that will give the best possible analytical results',[9] that is, the most accurate results. However, one can also have practical sensitive, reliable and specific methods that are suitable for routine use in the real-life environment[9] of a service laboratory. Such routine methods will probably have some bias in relation to the reference method.

This is probably the best place at which to emphasize the fact that the consensus value of a number of methods for any substance does not necessarily represent the 'true' value. Certainly the most precise method does not necessarily give the 'true' value, although it may temporarily provide a useful reference point.

(b) 'Standardization discourages individual thought and the development of individual skill and satisfaction in work.'[10]

Of course this can be true, but it need not be true if those directing standardization projects act wisely. A properly co-ordinated study of a method can be expected to require the work of many people; this will be the case both initially and during periods when a method is being revised. For example, the Institute of Petroleum has for years had about 60 sub-groups engaged in keeping its methods up to date.

(c) Advantages of standardization include:

(i) As already mentioned, involvement of many workers, sharing the load of investigation of what may be a complex method.

(ii) Early criticism of proposed methods.

(iii) Early elimination of unsatisfactory methods. One can only guess at the immense amount of time which must have been wasted in the *unorganized* investigation of such methods.

6.7 STANDARDIZATION OF NEW TECHNIQUES

Even newer instrumental methods of analysis can be subjected to this approach. Egan[5] has pointed out that 'the results of early studies of this kind were, not unexpectedly, disappointing, especially when it is recalled that they were at the same time seeking to achieve levels of sensitivity and specificity which, until shortly beforehand, had been regarded as impossible. But these very considerations acted as a spur to reach acceptable standards in these new fields'.

Such a conclusion ought to encourage us to a closer, organized study of the methods used for estimation of the proteins which are being discussed at this symposium and should lead us to expect a successful outcome to such work.

References

1. Belk, W. P. and Sunderman, F. W. (1946). A survey of the accuracy of chemical analyses in clinical laboratories. *Am. J. Clin. Pathol.,* **17,** 853
2. Watson, D. and Pow, M. (1976). Diagnostic reagents for alpha-fetoprotein. *Lancet,* **i,** 1015
3. Cooper, G. R. (1968). Standardization and control of quantitative analyses. *Z. Anal. Chem.,* **243,** 816
4. Cali, J. P. (1973). An idea whose time has come. *Clin. Chem.,* **19,** 291
5. Egan, H. (1972). Collaborative analysis and the standardization of analytical methods. *Proc. Soc. Anal. Chem.,* **9,** 245
6. Griffiths, J. G. A. (1950). Foreword. In 'Standardization in the Chemical Field', *Lect. Monogr. Rep. R. Inst. Chem.,* No. 5
7. Johnson, W. C. and Osborn, G. H. (1950). Standardization in the chemical field. p. 10. *Lect. Monogr. Rep. R. Inst. Chem.,* No. 5
8. Expert Panel on Proteins (1976). News Letter No. 13. International Federation of Clinical Chemistry, p. 4
9. Rodgerson, D. O. and Tietz, N. W. (1975). Selection of 'recommended methods' for use in a clinical laboratory—some urgent considerations and a suggested approach. *Clin. Chem.,* **21,** 1057
10. Garratt, D. C. (1950). Standardization of methods of analysis. p. 16. *Lect. Monogr. Rep. R. Inst. Chem.,* No. 5

7

Quality control

D. M. Browning

7.1   INTRODUCTION   75

7.2   EXTERNAL QUALITY CONTROL   76

7.3   QUALITY CONTROL IN IMMUNOCHEMISTRY   79

7.4   CONCLUSIONS   80

7.1   INTRODUCTION

Quality control in its various forms has been an ever increasing activity in our clinical chemistry laboratories for more than two decades. Although there have been many publications over the years stating quite clearly how useful and profitable such activities are, some laboratory workers continue to question its usefulness and react emotionally to the philosophy and practice of quality control techniques. Quality control techniques should not be used with the objective of 'catching the laboratory worker out' but to help us to perform with a greater degree of reliability. It should be used to enhance the work of the laboratory.

We should perhaps remind ourselves what we really mean by the term quality control. In his book *Quality Control in Clinical Chemistry*, Professor Whitehead[1] defines it as 'The use of a variety of measures and techniques to reduce the variance in laboratory results'.

Quality control of course starts with the taking of a suitable specimen from a subject and ends with the transmission and recording of a result. The analytical procedure in between is subject to a measurable variance but the first and last stages are also subject to an often grossly underrated variance. The effect of stasis on many clinical chemistry determinations is well known but there is a measurable variance due to other non-analytical difficulties. The introduction of data handling, automated techniques, and computers have of course helped reduce errors due to the recording of results. Most of our attempts to monitor the performance of tests have concentrated on the analytical variance which is more easily measured and controlled.

All laboratory workers perform some form of quality control, although they may not recognise it as such. We all use some standard or reference material for comparative purposes. Although we may not carry out a specific quality control determination we will invariably carry out a subjective assessment of our results. Are they all too high or too low? Why is it that in a large batch there are no abnormals? These subjective assessments are being replaced by judgements based on scientific evidence. A variety of methods for assessing the precision and accuracy of test results are available to us. All are useful but it can be demonstrated that internal quality control systems can be designed to give comfort rather than challenge. It is important that we continuously challenge all our methods and techniques, and quality control techniques are no exception.

7.2   EXTERNAL QUALITY CONTROL

Since 1969 in the UK we have developed a philosophy of challenge by using the technique of external quality control. Such techniques have become an integral part of laboratory life and there can be very few laboratory workers who are not challenged by it. We can show that the use of this technique of inter-laboratory challenge enables us to assess methods, measure performance and take collective action so that we begin to perform in a more acceptable way. The method inevitably involves the use of consensus values.

Figures 7.1 and 7.2 show how the urea results from two laboratories compare with the results achieved over a period of time on the National Quality Control Scheme. Both laboratories use a diacetyl monoxime method on the AutoAnalyser. One laboratory produces results consistently closer to

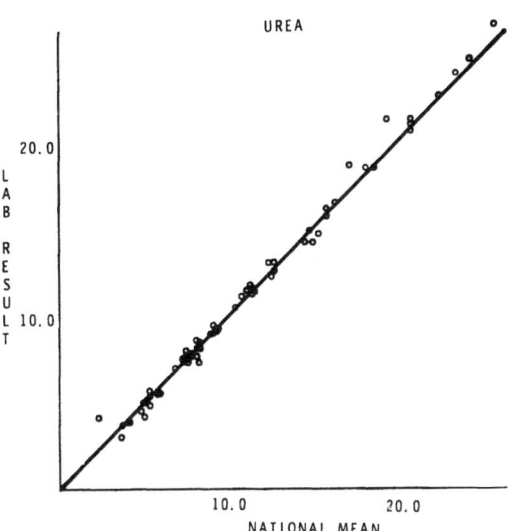

Figure 7.1 Cumulative relationship of laboratory A to national mean, NQCS urea determinations

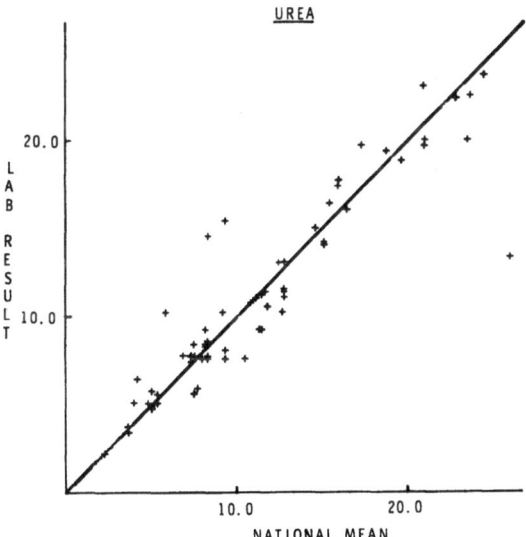

Figure 7.2 Cumulative relationship of laboratory B to national mean, NQCS urea determinations

the national mean, the other shows results which are much more variable. Similar results can be demonstrated for most determinations currently being surveyed in the National Quality Control Scheme.

Using this technique of external quality control we have been able to measure the overall performance of laboratories using the calculation of the Variance Index[2]. This is defined as the difference between the result obtained and the correct value, expressed at a percentage of the correct value, divided by a chosen coefficient of variation for that determination; the resultant figure is multiplied by 100. It is calculated in the following way: The method mean (X_m) is subtracted from the result of an individual laboratory (X), and the percentage variation (V) from the method mean is calculated:

$$\frac{V = X - X_m}{X_m} \times 100$$

The variance index (VI) is calculated from this figure by dividing it by the chosen coefficient of variation (CCV). This figure is multiplied by 100:

$$VI = \frac{V}{CCV} \times 100$$

Using the mathematical expression we have been able to demonstrate the usefulness of external quality control systems. Figure 7.3 shows how the Mean Running Variance Index Score may be plotted to demonstrate changes in the overall performance of a laboratory. Publicizing this information to participants has enabled us to demonstrate the degree of improvement that can occur. Significant factors may well be the changes that have taken place in the methods in use in the UK. Manual methods for many of our routine

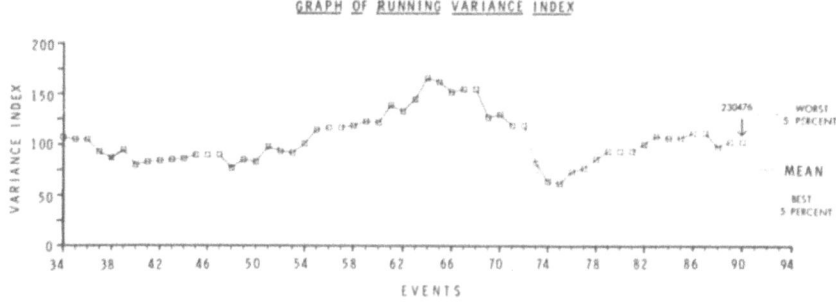

Figure 7.3   Serial plot of Mean Running Variance Index Score

determinations have been replaced by automated techniques or improved chemical methods. Total protein and albumin determinations are examples. In the former, we have eliminated the specific gravity method; whilst in the latter the BCG method for albumin, although not without its problems, has at least enabled us to improve the precision of our test results. Few laboratories now persist in using the salt fractionation methods which are notorious for the difficulties which are experienced when one attempts to achieve precise results.

7.3   QUALITY CONTROL IN IMMUNOCHEMISTRY

These established techniques are fine for routine clinical chemistry, but what is the situation in the specific protein and immunochemistry fields? The information is a good deal more limited. However, Figure 7.4 shows the results from three laboratories participating in an inter-laboratory quality control scheme for IgA. The results over a period of time are plotted as a percentage deviation from the overall mean. The three sets of results are confusing because of the confusion in the data caused by obvious standardization problems. In Figure 7.5 the same data is plotted after each set of results have

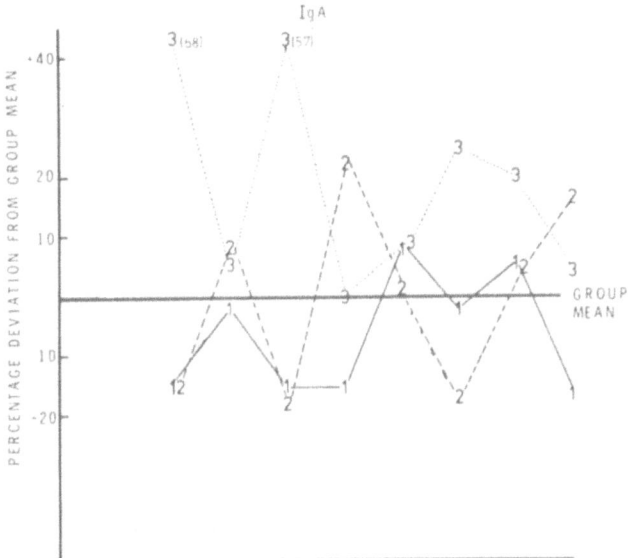

Figure 7.4   Inter-laboratory quality control scheme for IgA. Percentage deviations from the group mean for three laboratories (1, 2, 3)

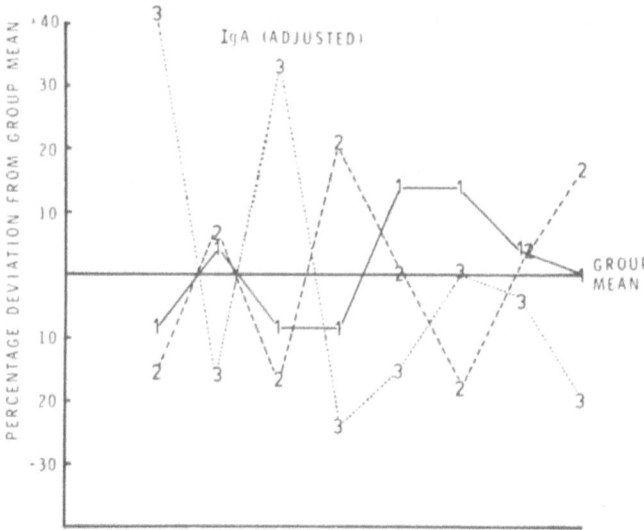

Figure 7.5 Same data as Figure 7.4 adjusted for differences in primary standard

been 'adjusted' for the accuracy differences in the laboratory. Laboratory 1 now has results which are close to the mean and evenly distributed either side of the group mean value. Laboratory 2 has results which have not been affected by the adjustment. Although the results are evenly distributed either side of the mean there is considerable deviation from the mean. Laboratory 3 has results which are not only high but also demonstrate very poor precision.

7.4 CONCLUSIONS

I believe I have demonstrated that the difficulties of accuracy and precision in protein immunochemistry are very similar to those that we have traditionally had with routine clinical chemistry tests. These difficulties still remain to some extent with, for example, cholesterol and enzyme determinations. I do not believe that a defensive statement to the effect that immunochemistry determinations are different can be justified. It has to be admitted that the use of consensus testing methods does have a limited value where there are difficulties in standardization due to the availability or willingness to use a suitable reference material. Nevertheless, we must not allow this to justify the continued production of results from various laboratories that cannot be compared with one another.

References

1. Whitehead, T. P. (1977). *Quality Control in Clinical Chemistry,* p. 125. (New York: John Wiley)
2. Whitehead, T. P., Browning, D. M., and Gregory, A. (1976). The role of external quality control schemes in improving the quality of laboratory results. *Quality Control in Clinical Chemistry (Transactions of the VIth International Symposium).* (Berlin: Walter de Gruyler)

SECTION TWO

Specific Proteins in Laboratory Diagnosis

Chairmen: Mr D. M. Browning,
Dr R. S. H. Pumphrey, Dr J. Kohn,
Professor J. Hardwicke and
Dr A. C. Munro

SECTION TWO

Specific Proteins in
Laboratory Diagnosis

8

Structure and function of the immunoglobulins
R. S. H. Pumphrey

8.1 INTRODUCTION   85

8.2 STRUCTURE   86

8.3 FUNCTION   88
    8.3.1 *Antigen binding*   88
    8.3.2 *The hinge region*   89
    8.3.3 *Effector and control functions*   92
        8.3.3.1 *IgM*   92
        8.3.3.2 *IgD*   94
        8.3.3.3 *IgG*   94
        8.3.3.4 *IgA*   95
        8.3.3.5 *IgE*   96

8.1 INTRODUCTION

The structure and function of immunoglobulins is so frequently reviewed that there is no point in providing multiple references in a short discussion such as this. Instead, a very few references are given at the end to give an introduction to the literature.

8.2 STRUCTURE

Immunoglobulins are built from heavy and light chains assembled in pairs (Figure 8.2). The light chains have two domains, the heavy three, four or five, according to class. Each domain has 110–120 amino acids, and all domains have a very similar structure (Figure 8.3), comprising two layers of anti-parallel β-pleated sheet. This makes a box with two faces (the X with four strands, the Y with three) held together by its hydrophobic interior, and stabilized by a disulphide bridge between the two faces. In the parts of the chain making up the β-pleated sheet, there is a very high degree of uniformity between all the different domains, but there is very little homology in those parts that form the bends between the β-pleated strands. The N-terminal domains of both heavy and light chains are called the variable (V) regions and differ from the remaining constant (C) domains by having a few extra amino acids near the mid-point of the domain. The domains can pair up by non-covalent forces, between the Y faces for the V domains, the X faces for the C domains. The heavy and light chains are further held together by disulphide bridges between the chains (Figures 8.2 and 8.4). There are oligo-saccharide side-chains at strategic points which modify the way in which adjacent domains interact.

There are five classes of serum immunoglobulin: IgM, IgD, IgG, IgA, and IgE, which differ by their heavy chains; these are μ, δ, γ, α and ε respectively. Subclasses may be distinguished, as for example in the human IgG$_1$ IgG$_2$, IgG$_3$ and IgG$_4$, with γ_1, γ_2, γ_3 and γ_4 heavy chains. Each subclass is found with both κ and λ light chains and the ratio of κ is a charac-teristic of each subclass.

Each subclass is represented by a single gene. All the heavy-chain C-region genes are in a single unit, with their associated V-region genes at one end of the complex (Figure 8.5). There are at least three basic types of heavy-chain V-region genes: V_{HI}, V_{HII} and V_{HIII}. The light-chain genes are completely separate, with V and C in one linkage group, V_λ and C_λ in another (Figure 8.5).

Two classes of immunoglobulin, IgM and IgA, have an extra 19 C-terminal amino acids in the last C_H domain, which enable them to polymerize in the presence of a different peptide made by the plasma cells, called the J chain: IgM to a pentamer, IgA to a dimer or tetramer of the unit structure (Figures 8.1 and 8.4). In secretions these higher order polymers are mostly bound to 'secretor piece', a protein made in epithelial cells.

There are five domains in the heavy chains of IgM and IgE. The other classes in humans have four domains; in these the two N-terminal domains (V_H and C_H1) are separated from the two C-terminal domains by a sequence of amino acids called the 'hinge' region, which takes the place of the fifth domain. In all classes V_H and $C_H 1$ pair up with the two light-chain domains, V_L and C_L, to form the 'Fab' (fragment with antibody activity). The two C-terminal domains of the heavy chain are called the Fc (fragment which crystallizes; the names derive from the properties of papain digests of rabbit IgG).

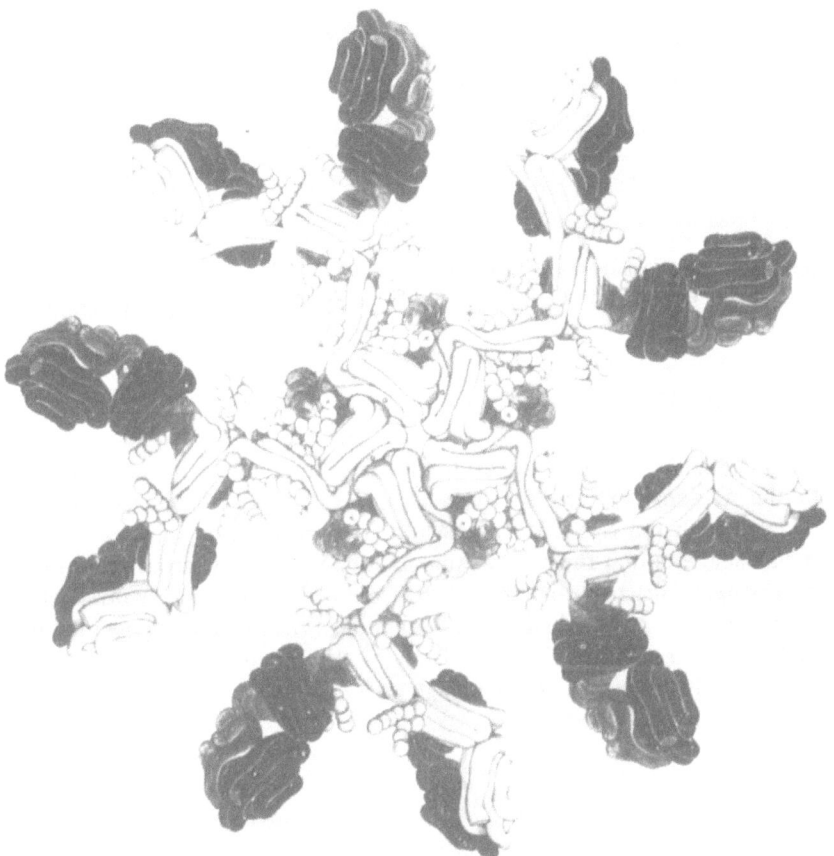

Figure 8.1 Model of an IgM molecule. The heavy chains are white and grey, the light chains black. The configuration of the oligosaccharide side-chains (shown as strings of spheres) and of the 19 C-terminal amino acids are speculative. It is possible that the C-terminal tail can take up quite different positions in the three forms of IgM: membrane monomer, serum monomer and serum pentamer. (Unfortunately during preparation of this illustration the C-terminal oligosaccharide has become misplaced, and its first N-acetylglucosamine, marked x, should be attached to an asparagine in the C-terminal tail, marked o)

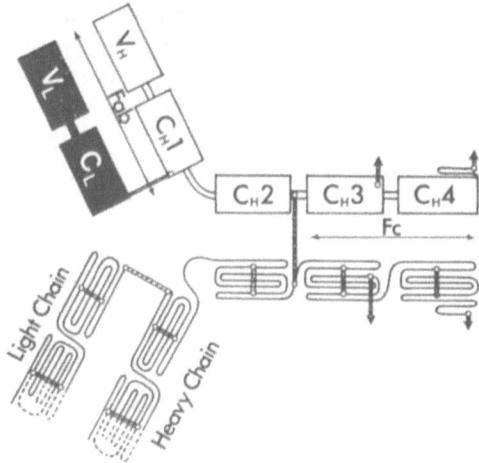

Figure 8.2 Block diagram of one IgM subunit. The discontinuous lines in the V-domains in the lower half of the diagram mark the hypervariable regions

8.3   FUNCTION

Immunoglobulins have two aspects to their function: antigen binding associated with the V domains, and a multiplicity of effector and control functions associated with the rest of the molecule. The structure of repeating similar domains suggests that the whole immunoglobulin molecule arose in evolution from a single ancestral domain. Since then, each domain has evolved along its own lines, and acquired specialized functions. The function of any immunoglobulin however, differs from the sum of the functions of its component domains, as much depends on the hinge region, which controls the interaction between the F ab and the Fc.

8.3.1   Antigen binding

Where the V_H and V_L domains meet, there is a site where antigens bind (Figure 8.6). It is formed by the loops at the N-terminal end of the domain. The rest of the V domain has a relatively constant structure, but these loops round the antigen binding site are 'hypervariable'.

Antibodies are secreted by plasma cells, which are the end-product of a long line of cell types. At the start of the line comes the B-lymphocyte stem-cell. This cell seems able to modify its chromosomal DNA in a way which is unique in our present understanding of genetics: starting with a small basic library of V-region genes, it selects one from the light-chain part of the library, and one from the heavy-chain part. It then randomly generates one of many (? about 10^4) possible sequences from each. For the greater part of their length these have the same sequence as the germ-line gene from which they started, but they differ in just those parts which code for the loops of the amino-acid chain round the binding site.

There is an alternative explanation for the generation of diversity among the many possible binding sites. This supposes that the diversity arose on the phylogenic time-scale, not the ontogenic; in other words the higher mammals have evolved a vast library of V-region genes, and the B-lymphocyte stem-cell merely has to select one gene from each of the heavy- and light-chain parts of the library.

At the end of this process, the light-chain V-region gene is expressed with its appropriate C-region gene, and the heavy-chain V-region gene with its μ C-region gene. This IgM is synthesized and appears on the cytoplasmic membrane of the B-cell. Each binding site structure may be expected to bind to several antigens, with a certain affinity for each. Following an antigenic stimulus, the immune response matures with selection of those cells whose membrane IgM binds most strongly to the antigen. These selected cells then secrete antibody with this defined antigen binding site, but can modulate the function of the antibody by changing the constant part of the heavy chain (see below). During this process the light-chain type remains unchanged: there seems to be little difference in the function of antibodies with κ or λ light chains.

An essential feature of this process is the transcription of the mRNAs from which the protein chain is synthesized from two separated sequences in the chromosomal DNA. It used to be thought that this was unique to immuno-globulins, but recent advances in the understanding of protein synthesis indicate that it may happen for most proteins made by eukaryotic cells.

8.3.2 The hinge region

The structure of the hinge region varies greatly between the classes and sub-classes of immunoglobulin (Figure 8.4). It contains one or more half-cystines (involved in interchain disulphide bridges) and is comparatively rich in proline. It is thought to be extended in IgG_3 and IgD, with up to fifteen half-cystines in IgG_3. In IgG_2 and IgG_4 it allows the Fab less freedom of movement which may make the Fab obscure the C1q binding site on the C_H2 domain even after it has bound to antigen. (Intact IgG_4 does not bind to C1q, but its Fc can, suggesting that the binding site is present but masked in the whole molecule.) In IgM and IgE, which do not have a special hinge region sequence, the extra domain acts as the mechanical link between Fab and Fc. No special functions have as yet been defined for this extra domain.

When the Fab end has bound to antigen, a number of changes must occur at the Fc end. The simplest change is the aggregation of several Fc's when their respective Fab's bind to multivalent antigen. If the Fc's are held by Fc receptors on the cytoplasmic membrane of a cell, the close-packed raft of Fc receptors which results may trigger one of several cellular functions (e.g. differentiation to antibody production for B-lymphocytes, release of histamine

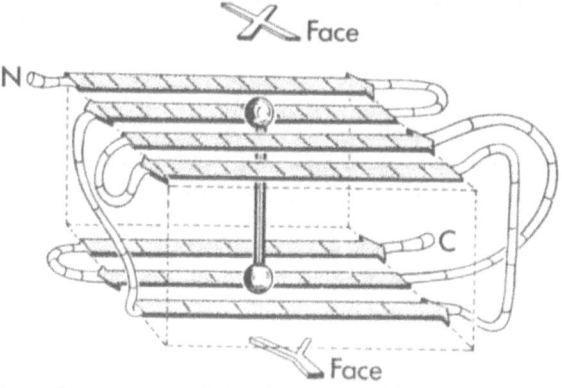

Figure 8.3 Schematic structure of the domain. In fact the structure is somewhat twisted, and the strands of the β-pleated sheet in the foreground are only half the length of those near the N- and C-terminal ends of the domain

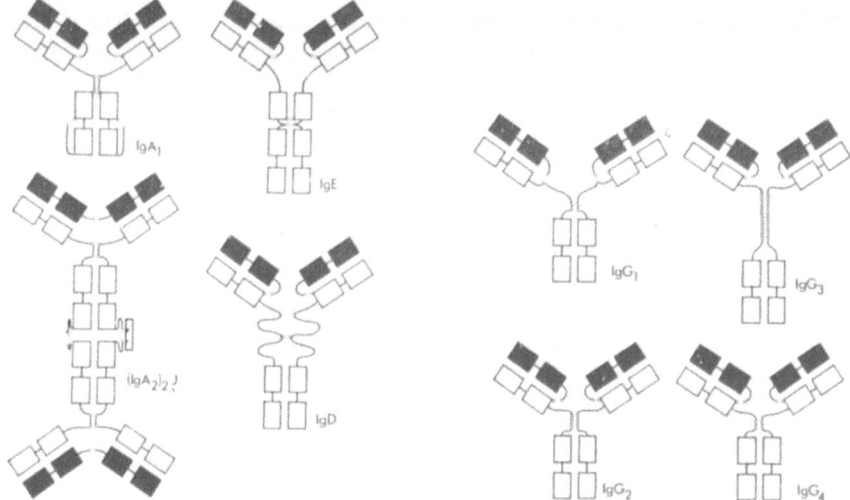

Figure 8.4 Block diagrams of the domains, hinge regions, and inter-chain disulphide bridges. (The cystines are shown as close pairs of open circles.)

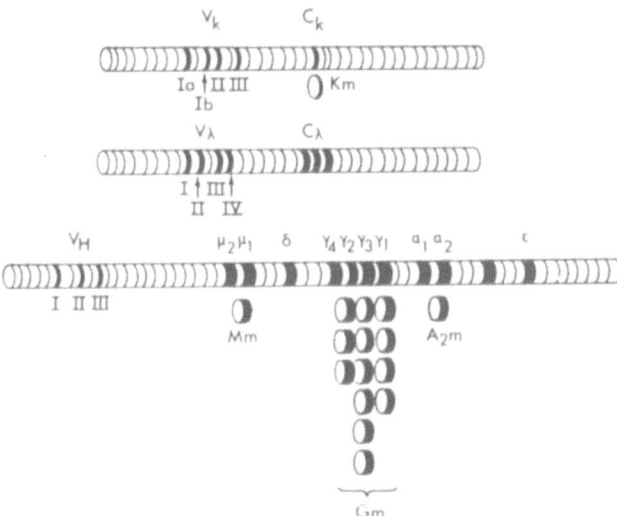

Figure 8.5 The three linkage groups of genes involved in synthesis of the immuno-globulin polypeptide chains. The allotypes are represented as discs which can insert as alternatives in the column of genes. The order of the genes in each linkage group is not known, and the number of V-region genes shown is the minimum possible. There *may* be thousands of V-region genes

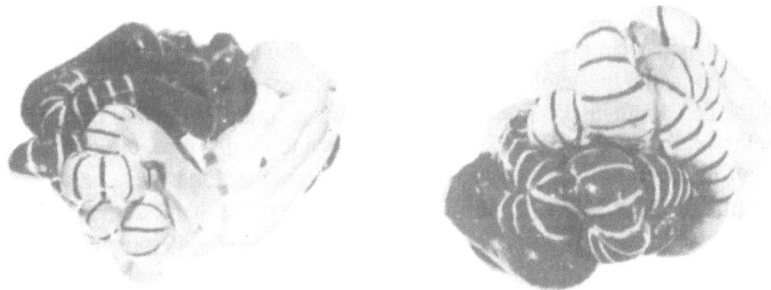

Figure 8.6 Model of the Fab, to show the extent of the binding site. The hyper-variable regions are shown by the white stripes

from mast cells, killing by K-cells, etc.). If the antibody molecules are free in solution before the Fab's bind, the clustering of Fc's may be enough to allow C1q to bind to the C_H2 of IgG, or it may be that the hinge region has to transmit a structural change from the bound Fab's to the Fc. The most drastic role suggested for the hinge region is in IgD, where the long hinge is exceptionally susceptible to enzymic lysis (e.g. by plasmin). Here it is suggested that antigen binding by the Fab may lead to enzymic cleavage of the hinge, and the effector function of the Fc or Fab then follows due to structural rearrangement or exposure of a new binding site.

8.3.3   Effector and control functions

The heavy chains have evolved to perform a wide variety of effector and control functions, which are most easily discussed by taking each class in turn. The heavy chain expressed with the antigen binding site is always μ in the earliest B-cells. Later IgM may be present on the surface of the B-lymphocyte in combination with IgD or one of the other classes, or IgM, IgD, and one of the other classes all together. The exact sequence of events and the role of the IgD is still controversial. The final class of immunoglobulin varies with the type and route of antigenic stimulation, and depends on genetic and constitutional factors in the responder.

8.3.3.1   IgM

IgM is the most primitive immunoglobulin, and the least specialized. It was the first to appear in the evolution of the vertebrates; it is the first to appear in the fetal development of vertebrates with more than one class of immunoglobulin; and it is the first to appear in any individual immune response.

When monomeric IgM first appears on the surface of B-cells, it gives the signal for further differentiation when it binds to antigen under the right conditions. These conditions seem to involve the proximity of macrophages (or rather, one of several cell types within the reticulo-endothelial system), and T-lymphocytes reacting to different determinants on the same antigen. At this early stage in the B-cell's development it can respond positively to a few types of antigen in the absence of T-cells (T-independent antigens) but it may respond negatively (become tolerized) to many stimuli.

As a membrane receptor IgM is monomeric, but most of the serum IgM is pentameric (Figure 8.1). Its ten binding sites allow for an avid antibody with comparatively low affinity at each site, but its large size hampers its access to extravascular antigen. Perhaps it was the development of higher affinity

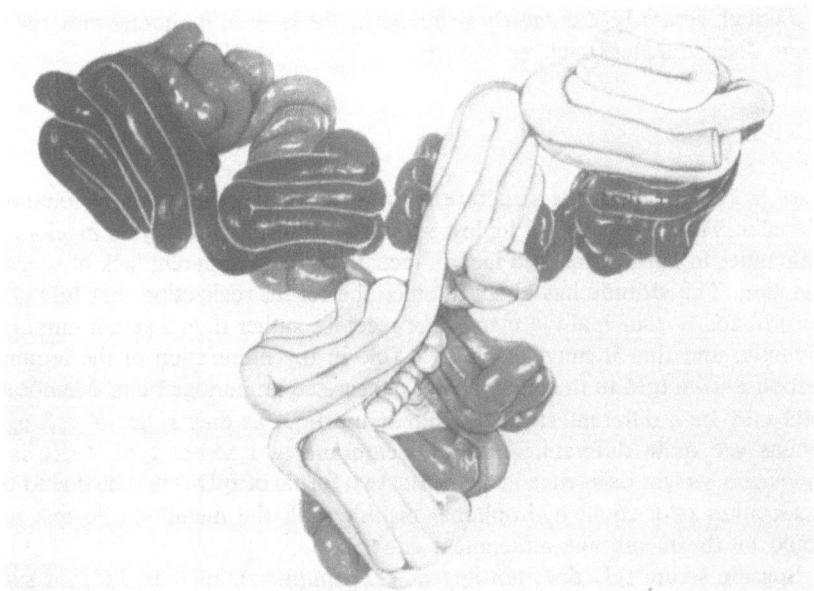

Figure 8.7 Model of an IgG molecule. The shades are as for Figure 8.1. The oligosaccharide side-chains are shown in the position they take in a crystal of an IgG$_1$ myeloma protein. In solution they may be free to float out like some of the oligosaccharides shown on the IgM model

antigen-binding sites which enabled the smaller monomeric immunoglobulins to succeed. The first monomeric immunoglobulins in evolution were probably IgM-like, with four C$_H$ domains, but there has been a trend to reduce the number of C$_H$ domains, producing smaller and more quickly diffusing molecules, first IgG-like with three C$_H$ domains, then IgM-like with two. (This type is found in some fishes, amphibia, reptiles, birds, and mammals, but not in man.)

IgM is an effective complement activating agent, and a single molecule bound to a red cell can initiate lysis *via* the classical pathway. (This requires multiple attachment of the IgM antibody. If the antigenic determinants are far-spaced, such as the Rhesus D antigen on red cells, the IgM can cause agglutination without fixing complement.) It is a good agglutinin with its multiple binding sites, though it is a poor opsonin in its own right, working principally through C3. It is not transmitted across the placenta from maternal to fetal circulation, which is important in preventing haemolytic disease of the newborn due to 'natural' anti-A or anti-B ABO blood group substance.

Though serum IgM is mostly pentameric, the level of monomer may rise in some disease states, such as in SLE.

8.3.3.2 IgD

Less is known about the structure of IgD than any other class of immuno-globulin. This is because of its low serum concentration, rarity of myelomas, difficulties in purification and lack of incentive due to apparent lack of specific function. The attitude has changed since the recent realization that IgD is in all probability principally a membrane receptor rather than a serum immuno-globulin, and that it may play a vital role in the maturation of the immune response from IgM to the other classes of secreted immunoglobulin. Membrane IgD may be a different subclass from serum IgD, as their ratios of $\kappa : \lambda$ light chains are quite different. As with membrane and serum IgM, there is a molecular weight difference between the two forms of IgD — maybe due to the association of a small hydrophobic peptide with the membrane forms; this could be the membrane attachment site.

Specific serum IgD does not appear after immunization with antigens such as tetanus toxoid. IgD auto-antibodies have, however, been found, though no specific function has been associated with IgD. Perhaps its role is to compete with other classes, and so block their action.

8.3.3.3 IgG

The evolution of immunoglobulins is rapid compared to some other proteins studied. The four human subclasses of IgG arose from an IgG_2-like precursor quite recently (only 10 million years ago, when the great apes were diverging from the other higher primates). Most other higher mammals have evolved specialized subclasses of IgG, such as the cow, where one subclass seems to be replacing IgA as the most important secretory immunoglobulin, and the guinea pig, where one subclass plays an IgE-like role (as indeed IgG can in man, though which subclass is not clear).

IgG is the principal serum immunoglobulin. More prolonged antigenic stimulation is required than for the IgM response, and co-operation with T cells is obligatory. (Thus one can recognize two phases to the humoral immune response: in the primary phase all the antibodies are IgM, in the secondary, IgG becomes the predominant class. This is because of the time taken for the B-cells to mature following their first encounter with the antigen, and their need for a second encounter before some of them are induced to become IgG-secreting plasma cells.)

In humans the secondary immune response to most protein antigens produces all four subclasses, roughly in proportion to their serum concentrations. Some antigens, however, produce subclass-restricted responses: anti-D of the Rhesus blood group system is usually IgG_1 and IgG_3, anti-factor VIII of the blood-clotting cascade and anti-grass pollen have been found to be IgG_4, and anti-dextran, IgG_2. It is not known what controls the production of a subclass-specific response, but it may well be due to the way the 'macrophage' and T cell present the antigen to the maturing B cell. Perhaps a tertiary stimulus is required to induce the B cell to mature beyond IgG_2 (the principal subclass on the surface of circulating B cells) to the other IgG subclasses.

The subclasses of IgG also differ in their function. While there is a very high degree of homology within the domains (around 90%), the hinge regions differ significantly. IgG_2 and IgG_4 have a hinge region which holds the Fab closer to the C_H2, so that even after antigen binding they cannot readily bind to C1q. This, of course, will not necessarily prevent them from activating complement by the alternative pathway (probably through the C_H1 domain), and so may not be such an important difference as it is usually made out to be.

Probably more important is the difference in binding to Fc receptors. IgG_1 and IgG_3 bind firmly to the Fc receptor on phagocytic cells, and have become an important trigger for these cells to 'internalize' material bound to their membranes. These subclasses are also probably the important ones for activating K cells. Crossing the placenta to the fetal circulation involves an active transport system, which also binds to the Fc, and is IgG_1 and IgG_3 specific.

Most immunoglobulins have a serum half-life of 3–8 days, but IgG_1, IgG_2, and IgG_4 are much longer lived, with half-lives of about 3 weeks. This, together with the selective transport, means that IgG_1 is the main subclass involved in passive immunization of the newborn, which has to last for about 3 months, until the baby starts to produce its own IgG.

IgG may also play an important part in the control of the immune response. When the level of serum IgG is high, there seems to be feedback suppression of all immunoglobulin synthesis. This can lead to a secondary humoral immunodeficiency in IgG myeloma.

8.3.3.4 IgA

IgA is the principal secretory immunoglobulin. In humans there is a considerable concentration in the serum (around 2–3 g/l, as opposed to 1–2 g/l for IgM, and 8–16 g/l for IgG) but this is mostly IgA_1 subclass, and mostly monomeric. It is not clear what its function is; it is not impossible that the serum IgA is just a scrap-heap of molecules which fail to get transported into the secretions.

It is, however, equally possible that monomeric IgA is evolving IgG-like functions in the human, in the same way that guinea pig IgG_1 has evolved some IgE-like activity, and IgG_1 in cows IgA-like activity.

The plasma cells making IgA are mostly close to the sites where it is secreted. Thus one finds numerous plasma cells around the collecting ductule in the lobules of the mammary gland, and in the lamina propria of the gut.

The dimeric form of IgA can bind to secretor piece, which is made by cells on many epithelial surfaces. Most of the IgA in the secretions is in the form $(IgA)_2.J.S.$ In this form it is much more resistant to enzymic attack than any any other class of immunoglobulin, which is useful for an antibody which has to function in a soup of digestive enzymes.

As its site of secretion might suggest, IgA production is best stimulated by the mucosal route of immunization, and best by live viruses or bacteria. The IgA response is early to mature, with virtually none in the saliva at birth, but rising to near adult levels by the age of 3 weeks. (The serum IgA appears much later.) Late development of secretory IgA is found in some infants that are failing to thrive. The concentration of secretor piece in the saliva is highest at birth, and falls after the appearance of the IgA.

In many species of mammal the transfer of IgA from mother to young through colostrum or milk seems to be very important in protecting the young. This may not only be relevant to bacteria and viruses, such as the transmissible gastro-enteritis virus in pigs, but also with food antigens, which can lead to a coeliac-like state in some young animals raised on artificial foods. There seems to be a special mechanism for attracting into the mammary gland those pre-plasma cells which normally recirculate to the gut. Thus the gut of the neonate is protected by the same antibodies as the gut of its mother.

IgA can activate complement via the alternative pathway, but not the classical. The level of complement in the secretions where IgA seems to be playing its major role is not high enough to suggest that this is really relevant to its mode of action. Probably it works against bacteria and viruses mainly by inhibiting their attachment to the mucosa, by blocking their binding sites. This mechanism seems to be much less effective in the absence of the normal commensal gut flora. It is not clear how important the antibody activity against food antigens is in preventing food allergy.

8.3.3.5   IgE

IgE is a cell surface receptor. It is only present in serum in transit from the IgE plasma cell to the mast cells and basophils, where it functions in conjunction with a specialized Fc receptor. The binding between the Fc of IgE and this receptor is exceptionally firm, and the low normal level of IgE is enough to 'top up' any newly synthesized Fc receptors on the histamine-secreting cells. Thus while each IgE plasma cell makes antibody with a single specificity, each histamine-secreting cell is coated with a film of IgE, with very many antibody specificities represented. In this membrane bound form, the IgE is relatively long-lived, with a half-life of about a fortnight, compared to its serum half-life of about 3 days.

When antigen binds with the membrane-bound IgE, histamine is secreted very rapidly, followed by a variety of other mediators. In the skin this causes the 'wheal and flare' reaction of type I hypersensitivity; in the mucosa one of the most important results is the increase in mucus production. There is concurrent smooth muscle spasm. Together, these form a powerful protective mechanism, with IgA blocking the binding sites of the pathogen, and IgE flushing it away in a torrent of mucus.

Some people produce much higher levels of IgE than normal in their mucosal immune response. They are called 'atopics', and tend to suffer from hayfever, asthma, urticaria, and eczema as a result of their over-enthusiastic IgE responses. The mechanism of the disease in the case of atopic eczema is far from clear; it certainly must differ from the local release of histamine and other mediators which causes atopic urticaria.

Despite the extreme rarity of IgE myelomas, the structure of IgE is known in considerable detail. The ε-chain has five domains with no special hinge region, like IgM, but it lacks the 19 C-terminal residues of IgM which are needed for polymerization. The C-terminal half of the molecule is heat-labile, and this has been used to distinguish IgE and IgG histamine-releasing antibodies. It is not known to activate complement or bind to phagocyte Fc receptors.

Bibliography

Nisonoff, A., Hopper, J. E. and Spring, S. B. (1975). *The Antibody Molecule.* (New York: Academic Press)

Feinstein, A. and Beale, D. (1978). Models of immunoglobulins and antigen–antibody complexes. In: M. Steward and L. E. Glynn (eds.). *Immunochemistry: an Advanced Textbook,* pp. 263–306 (Oxford: Blackwell Scientific Publications)

Immunoglobulin D: structure, synthesis, membrane representation and function (1977). *Immunol. Rev.,* **37,** Ed. Moller

9

Immunoglobulins in blood transfusion

P. D. J. Holt

9.1 INTRODUCTION 100

9.2 ANTIGENS OF IMMUNOGLOBULINS 100
 9.2.1 Classification of the major types of antigenic variation of immunoglobulins 100
 9.2.2 Methods used to detect antigenic variation of immunoglobulins 101

9.3 THE ANTIGENIC DETERMINANTS OF IgG, IgA AND IgM IMMUNOGLOBULINS 102
 9.3.1 Isotypic antigens of IgG 102
 9.3.2 Allotype antigens of IgG 103
  9.3.2.1 Implications in transfusion reactions 104
  9.3.2.2 Implications in reagent production 104
  9.3.2.3 Allotypes as genetic markers 105
  9.3.2.4 Allotype preference in antibodies 105
 9.3.3 Antigens of IgA 105
  9.3.3.1 Anti-IgA antibodies 106
  9.3.3.2 Implications in transfusion reactions 107
  9.3.3.3 IgA deficiency in blood donors 108
 9.3.4 Antigens of IgM 109
 9.3.5 Isoallotypes and idiotypes 110
  9.3.5.1 Isoallotype antigens 110
  9.3.5.2 Idiotype antigens 110

9.1   INTRODUCTION

Immunoglobulins are the group of proteins comprising the antibodies and they are of fundamental importance to blood transfusion. The basic function of any antibody is to combine with antigen and it is the observations and deductions made from examining such antibody–antigen reactions which form the basis of blood group immunology. The therapeutic value of immuno-globulin preparations has long been known and with the increased use of plasmaphoresis it is now the responsibility of Blood Transfusion Centres to test for and to prepare specific immune antibodies such as prophylactic anti-Rh, anti-tetanus toxin and anti-$HB_S Ag$ antibody. It would be perfectly possible, therefore, to discuss the importance of immunoglobulins in blood transfusion in their role as anti-blood group antibodies or as therapeutic immunoglobulin fractions.

It is, however, another aspect of immunoglobulins that will be discussed here, namely the situation where immunoglobulins themselves react as antigens in a specific antigen–antibody reaction. IgG, IgA and IgM immunoglobulins are the most important antigenically in blood transfusion. Fortunately, they are found in the highest concentrations in serum and so are easier to study. The major antigenic differences of these immunoglobulins and their signifi-cance in blood transfusion will be discussed.

9.2   ANTIGENS OF IMMUNOGLOBULINS

9.2.1   Classification of the major types of antigenic variation of immunoglobulins

The antigenic variation of the major immunoglobulin classes falls into four categories:

(a) *Isotype*—The isotype is the antigen or antigens which distinguish one class or subclass of immunoglobulin from another. For example if an experi-mental animal were immunized with a single immunoglobulin class the antibody produced would be directed principally to the isotype antigens and thus the antibody would not react with immunoglobulin of a different class.

(b) *Allotype*—Allotypes are antigens or genetic markers found on certain immunoglobulin heavy or light chains, the expression of which is controlled by polymorphic genes. It has been shown in many cases [1-3] that the allotypic variation of immunoglobulins is due to one or two amino-acid substitutions within the constant region of the appropriate heavy or light chains.

(c) *Isoallotype*—Isoallotypes are a series of antigenic determinants originally described as non-markers. They occur as allotypes within a subclass and as isotypes on one or more of the remaining sub-classes.

(d) *Idiotype*—Idiotype antigens confer a certain uniqueness to immunoglobulin molecules and are determined by certain areas of the variable region of the heavy and light chains. An anti-idiotype antibody will usually block the antibody-combining site of an immunoglobulin molecule when reacted with it.

9.2.2 Methods used to detect antigenic variation of immunoglobulins

One of the principal methods for detecting the reaction between soluble antigen and its corresponding antibody is immunoprecipitation. This method, however, has requirements for large amounts of antigen and a strong antibody. The reactions of many of the antibodies to immunoglobulins do not very often fulfil the criteria required for immunoprecipitation, and for this reason the system most commonly used in the investigation of the reactions of anti-immunoglobulin is passive haemagglutination (PHA) and inhibition of passive haemagglutination (PHAI).

In many circumstances in the study of the allotypic antigens of IgG (Gm and Km antigens) use is made of the specificity of certain immune anti-blood group antibodies for red cells. These are selected for their ability to sensitize cells with appropriate Gm or Km antigen. The most common system used is rhesus positive red cells sensitized with incomplete anti-rhesus antibody. In other cases the antigen is usually purified monoclonal immunoglobulin protein and is coupled to red cells chemically using chromic chloride or tannic acid.

One consequence of the use of Rhesus sensitized cells for the study of anti-IgG antibodies is that the combination of the IgG anti-Rhesus antibody with the erythrocyte surface causes the immunoglobulin to undergo conformational change, and this in turn leads to the exposure of new antigenic receptors. Thus there are many anti-antibodies which react with Rh coated cells but are not inhibited by the antigen in the free state. There is a similar problem when using purified monoclonal proteins but this is usually due to denaturation of the immunoglobulin by incorrect storage conditions.

9.3   THE ANTIGENIC DETERMINANTS OF IgG, IgA AND IgM IMMUNOGLOBULINS

9.3.1   Isotypic antigens of IgG

Human IgG consists of four major subclasses (Figure 9.1). Each subclass has an isotype antigen which distinguishes it from other subclasses, and in addition each has isotype antigens which contribute towards the overall antigenicity of IgG.

IgG immunoglobulins are, of course, extremely important in blood transfusion, the majority of clinically significant antibodies being of this class. When considering the significance of IgG isotypes in blood transfusion one must include the role that anti-isotype antibodies have. One of the most important laboratory tests in blood group serology is the Coombs test. This test is based on the reaction of anti-isotype antibodies, raised in experimental animals, with immunoglobulin coating the target red cells. This constitutes a prime example of the value of isotype antigens, for without them this reaction would not be possible. An extension of the Coombs test is to use antisera specific for the sub-classes of IgG. It is somewhat unfortunate that these antisera are particularly difficult to make, and thus the isotypic variation between the sub-classes cannot be all that great. It has been shown that many anti-blood group antibodies are IgG_1 and IgG_3[4]. It is possible that investigation of the subclass of anti-blood group antibodies and the auto-antibodies that cause auto-immune haemolytic anaemia might yield potentially useful information on the clinical significance of such antibodies.

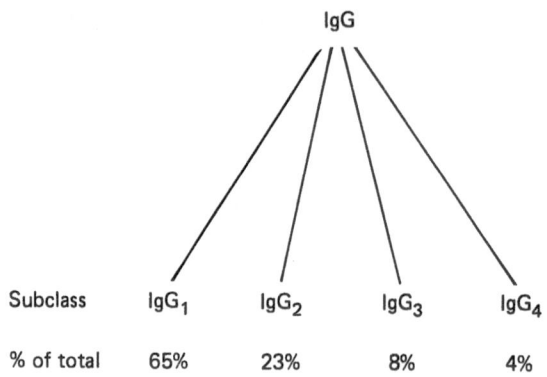

Figure 9.1   The subclasses of human IgG

With respect to human antibodies to isotypes of IgG it is difficult to conceive of the production of anti-class specific IgG in a patient, as a complete absence of IgG would be a necessary prerequisite for this. It is possible for a patient to produce antibodies to IgG derived from a phylogenetically distinct species, something that may in part be associated with the serum sickness often seen with the use of horse anti-tetanus or anti-diphtheria globulin.

Anti-IgG antibodies have long been observed in the sera of patients suffering from various immune complex diseases such as rheumatoid arthritis. It is thought that these antibodies consist of a number of different anti-immunoglobulins, including many that react with immunoglobulin that has been altered by immunological reaction and some that react as specific allotype antibodies[5,6].

9.3.2 Allotype antigens of IgG

The allotype antigens of IgG were first detected by Grubb[6]. Table 9.1 shows the distribution of the allotypes within the subclasses of IgG; the nomen-

TABLE 9.1   Allotypic markers of human IgG

Immunoglobulin subclass	Location	Allotypes		
IgG₁	Fc	G1m1		
		2		
	Fab(Fd)	G1m3		
		17		
IgG₂	Fc	G2m23		
IgG₃	Fc	G3m11	6	26
		5	24	27
		13	21	
		14	15	
		10	16	
IgG₄	—	none		
All	Kappa chain C-region	Km 1		
		2		
		3		

clature used is that which was proposed by a WHO meeting on human immunoglobulin allotype markers[7]. The majority of allotype antigens have been detected on subclasses IgG_1 and IgG_3, this is not really unexpected as the usual way of demonstrating IgG allotypes is with anti-Rhesus sensitized red cells and anti-Rhesus is usually either IgG_1 or IgG_3.

9.3.2.1 Implications in transfusion reactions

One of the major aspects of the significance of allotypic markers of IgG in blood transfusion is the question of whether the presence of an anti-allotype antibody will cause a transfusion reaction in a patient receiving blood. To answer this the origin of anti-allotype antibodies must first be considered.

There are three sources of anti-allotype antibodies:

(a) Normal patient sera (human non-rheumatoid arthritis sera)
(b) Rheumatoid arthritis sera
(c) Heteroimmune antisera.

Certain of the allotypic markers of IgG have been demonstrated only by heteroimmune antisera raised to purified monoclonal proteins so these may be ignored in this context. In the case of blood transfusions given to patients suffering from rheumatoid arthritis, it is not practice to screen this blood for compatible Gm allotypes. A great many transfusions will have been given to these patients without any apparent ill-effects, even in those possessing very powerful anti-allotype antibodies.

Transfusion reactions have been encountered in non-rheumatoid patients who have high titred anti-allotype antibodies[8]. It was concluded by van Loghem that the immunoglobulin class of the anti-allotype antibody may be more important than the target antigen. It would appear that IgG type antibodies may cause transfusion reactions whereas IgM antibodies do not.

9.3.2.2 Implications in reagent production

It is the policy of the United Kingdom Blood Group Reference Laboratory to reject any routine blood grouping antiserum that may be contaminated with anti-allotype antibodies. The reason for this policy is that there are many instances where a patient's red cells may be coated in vivo with IgG antibody, and it would therefore be dangerous to use a grouping antiserum which contains anti-allotype antibody with cells that may be coated with the respective allotype antigen. An example of this problem is described by Konugres[9] et al. who report the case of a patient whose red cells gave a strongly positive direct antiglobulin reaction, where an incorrect Rh group was determined due to the presence of contaminating anti-G1m2 reacting with the auto-antibody coating the cells.

9.3.2.3 Allotypes as genetic markers

The allotypes of IgG serve as very useful genetic markers in anthropological surveys and in the study of the phylogenetic origins of antibody molecules. Some of the more common allotypes are used in forensic serology for the identification of blood samples and stains and in the serological investigation of disputed paternity.

9.3.2.4 Allotype preference in antibodies

It is apparent that certain allotype antigens are preferentially expressed on some blood group antibodies, particularly anti-Rhesus antibodies. Litwin[10] analysed anti-Rhesus derived from individuals heterozygous for the G1m1 and G1m3 antigens and showed a marked shift towards the predominance of G1m1 anti-Rh. This would indicate that some form of selection within the IgG subclass is occurring. One has to be very careful when trying to interpret the significance of such observations, but one possible application may be in the selection of male volunteers for immunization with Rhesus antigen for the production of prophylactic anti-Rh. Would a G1m1 individual give a better response?

9.3.3 Antigens of IgA

IgA can be distinguished from IgG by virtue of the isotypic variation which contributes to the antigenicity of the immunoglobulin class. Whereas human IgG has been shown to consist of four major subclasses human IgA has only two subclasses, IgA_1 and IgA_2. In addition the subclass can be distinguished by isotypic antigens unique to either IgA_1 or IgA_2, this antigenic variation must in part be due to the quite profound configurational differences between the subclasses.

In addition to isotypic differences two allotype antigens are demonstrable on IgA (Figure 9.2) and one isoallotype has also been described. It is interesting to note that allotypes of IgA have only been demonstrated on IgA_2 and yet this subclass is the minor component of serum IgA, being only

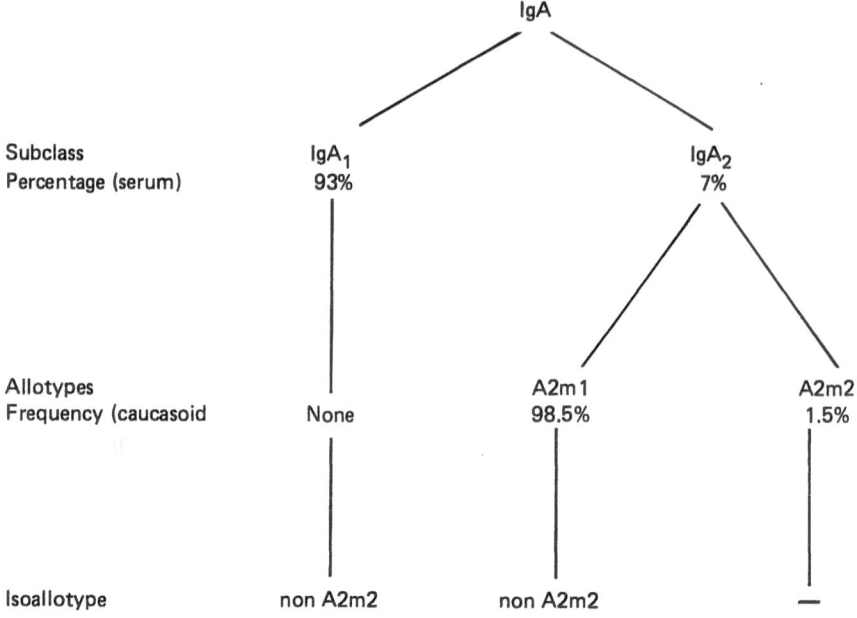

Figure 9.2   Subclasses and antigens of human IgA_1

7% of the total. This fact is still more surprising when one considers the manner in which the antigenic differences of IgA are demonstrated; it is practice to use panels of isolated monoclonal IgA couple to red cells, the majority of which will be of the IgA_1 subclass, and yet no allotypes have been demonstrated on IgA_1 to date.

9.3.3.1   Anti-IgA antibodies

In blood transfusion practice considerable importance is given to the clinical significance of the immunoglobulin class of anti-blood group antibodies. It would appear that antibodies of the IgA class do not play a significant role as anti-blood group antibodies; those that are described are often associated with auto-immune haemolytic anaemia and it is only very rarely that one meets a specific blood group antibody of the IgA class.

IgA is, however, extremely important when considering the immunoglobulins as antigens since anti-IgA antibodies have frequently been demonstrated. It has also been shown that the presence of anti-IgA antibodies in a patient can cause severe anaphylactic transfusion reactions, sometimes with fatal consequences.

Generally anti-IgA antibodies can be classified into two categories:

(a) *Class-specific anti-IgA*—These antibodies react with all IgA proteins regardless of subclass or allotype and can be thought of as true isotype antibodies reacting with the IgA immunoglobulin class. Class-specific antibodies are normally only found in individuals who have an immunodeficiency of IgA.

(b) *Anti-IgA of limited specificity*—The anti-IgA antibodies of limited specificity react with only selected IgA proteins. They can appear as isotype antibodies reacting with the subclass antigens of IgA_1 or IgA_2 or as allotypic antibodies reacting with the A2m1 or A2m2 antigens, or there may be a mixture of different specificities. Limited specificity antibodies can be present in individuals who have an immunodeficiency of IgA or in individuals with apparently normal IgA levels who lack either the subclass or the allotype towards which their antibody is directed.

9.3.3.2 Implications in transfusion reactions

Since the introduction of the passive haemagglutination technique using chromic chloride as a coupling agent with purified proteins, many laboratories have detected non-precipitating anti-IgA antibodies in patients who experienced severe anaphylactic transfusion reactions[11–14]. The well-established cases have shown that the majority of such reactions are caused by high-titre class-specific anti-IgA antibodies of the IgG immunoglobulin class. Exceptionally strong antibodies of limited specificity have also been implicated in severe anaphylactic transfusion reactions[11]. Reports indicate[12–15] that these antibodies require only very small amounts of IgA antigen to provoke a reaction; in one experiment[12] a donation of red cells washed twice with physiological saline contained enough residual IgA to cause a reaction in a patient with strong class-specific anti-IgA, and it was only after a further three washings that the blood donation was tolerated.

In addition to the reports of severe anaphylactic reactions due to high-titre anti-IgA antibodies many workers have described the presence of a high percentage of weak anti-IgA antibodies with limited specificity in patients experiencing less severe anaphylactoid or urticarial type transfusion reactions[15–17]. In almost all these instances the antibodies detected have reacted only weakly with a very small number of IgA proteins, and further investigations have shown them to be inhibited only by the autologous proteins and not by random donor sera. It is certainly questionable whether weak limited-specificity anti-IgA alone could be responsible for transfusion reactions; indeed one study[17] found a high incidence of such antibodies in the random donor population and these donations were apparently tolerated quite normally by recipients. My own experience with these rather nebulous antibodies suggests that their detection may reflect properties of the very sensitive system used to demonstrate anti-IgA antibodies rather than a valid reaction caused by an antibody of limited specificity. Such apparent weak anti-IgA antibody activity is not generally reproducible phenomenon. This may in part be due to minor differences in the efficiency of the coupling of individual IgA proteins to the cells for use in passive haemagglutination tests or to the occurrence of antibodies to denatured IgA. Koistinen and Leikola[16] have reported a high frequency of antibodies to denatured IgA occurring in serum samples from the random donor population. Improper storage of the purified IgA proteins used for coupling could therefore lead to the detection of such antibodies which are of little significance. In many of the reports by workers detecting weak anti-IgA antibodies of limited specificity the titres of these antibodies are often $\frac{1}{8}$ or less. Antibodies of such low strength must be viewed with a good deal of scepticism as the likelihood of getting a reliable inhibition result is low and such inhibition tests are essential for the confirmation of the true nature and specificity of any anti-immunoglobulin antibody.

Transfusion reactions caused by strong anti-IgA antibodies are rare, but in most instances they have been serious enough to induce many countries to establish registers of IgA-deficient blood donors.

9.3.3.3   *IgA deficiency in blood donors*

Selective IgA deficiency is the most common immunoglobulin deficiency encountered. It has been shown to be associated with a variety of disorders such as recurrent infections, gastrointestinal disturbances and autoimmune diseases. IgA deficiency has also been found in apparently healthy blood donors [18–23].

The results of a study of the frequency of IgA deficiency in blood donors performed at the South West Regional Transfusion Centre are shown in Table 9.2. It is clear from the data presented that true IgA deficiency is a little difficult to define. When using a reasonably sensitive screening test 85 samples were detected in this series as having abnormally low levels of IgA. Further investigation using more sensitive techniques enables classification of the IgA deficiency into two types: those donors with minute amounts of IgA in the serum and those having a complete absence of IgA. It would appear that the degree of IgA deficiency depends on the method used to detect it for if radioimmunoassay is employed still fewer donors are shown to be completely deficient.

TABLE 9.2 IgA deficiency in blood donors of the south-west region of England

	No. of samples	Frequency
Total samples tested	43 203	—
IgA deficient by the screening test ($<40\,\mu g\,IgA/cm^3$)	85	1:508
IgA deficient by haemagglutination inhibition ($<0.5\,\mu g\,IgA/cm^3$)	57	1:758
Very low level of IgA 0.5–40 $\mu g\,IgA/cm^3$)	28	1:1543

An interesting aspect of the study of IgA deficiency has been the observation that normal numbers of IgA-bearing B-cells can be detected[24]. This raises the possibility that IgA deficiency could be due to an impairment of T-cell function rather than a defect of IgA structural genes.

Both class-specific anti-IgA and anti-IgA of limited specificity can be detected in the serum of approximately 25% of IgA deficient donors. In the 85 samples detected in the screening of South West Regional blood donors 12 class-specific antibodies and 9 limited-specificity antibodies were demonstrated. The presence of these antibodies in blood donors poses interesting problems: firstly, the donors with strong class-specific antibodies would certainly be at risk if they required a blood transfusion and so should carry a special blood group card warning of the dangers of indiscriminate transfusion, and, secondly, a unit of whole blood possessing strong anti-IgA antibodies may cause unfavourable reactions in a recipient who has normal IgA levels and therefore the use of such blood for routine transfusion purposes should be limited.

9.3.4 Antigens of IgM

Unlike IgG or IgA immunoglobulins no clear-cut subclasses have been demonstrated for the IgM immunoglobulin class. Some workers[25-26] have been able to show a certain serological heterogeneity which suggests there are at least two subclasses for IgM, but it would appear that these serological differences are minor and probably due to slight amino-acid sequence differences rather than the somewhat profound structural differences found in IgG and IgA subclasses.

A single allotype antigen known as Mm1 has been described for IgM by Wells et al.[27] but its existence has yet to be satisfactorily confirmed by other workers.

Very little information is available regarding the significance of IgM antigens. In a study by Leikola et al.[28] anti-IgM antibodies were detected in 7.2% of patients given multiple transfusion but no correlation was found between the presence of antibodies and the transfusion reaction. At the Bristol Blood Transfusion Centre we have been screening transfusion reaction sera for the presence of antibodies to IgA, IgM and IgG (Gm) for a number of years. A number of anti-IgM antibodies have been encountered but these have usually reacted with only a limited number of IgM proteins and are generally weak. On further investigation using passive haemagglutination inhibition these antibodies are only inhibited by the autologous protein and not by random donor sera. It is therefore unlikely that the presence of such antibodies could cause a transfusion reaction but as a precautionary measure patients with anti-IgM antibodies received either washed or well-packed red cells if further transfusion was required.

9.3.5   Isoallotypes and idiotypes

9.3.5.1   Isoallotype antigens

Isoallotypes have now been described on IgG and IgA molecules and these antigens were first referred to as 'non'-markers. If one considers the isoallotype non-G1m1 of IgG the antigen was first characterized chemically by Frangione et al.[1], who demonstrated a certain amino-acid sequence in the CH3 region common to all G1m1-negative IgG_1, all IgG_2 and all IgG_3 proteins. Subsequently an antibody was developed by Natvig et al.[29] which enabled the non-G1m1 antigen to be demonstrated serologically. Antibodies defining the isoallotypes are relatively rare. They are usually produced in experimental animals although human antibodies are not unknown. The significance of the isoallotype antigens remains in the chemical analysis of immunoglobulins, in the investigation of the phylogeny of immunoglobulin polymorphism and in the anthropological investigation of different ethnic populations.

9.3.5.2   Idiotype antigens

The idiotype antigens are not well characterized like other antigens of immunoglobulins. They are, however, destined for much more attention in the future. One possible use of anti-idiotype antibodies would be in conjunction with the recent experiments on the production of monoclonal antibodies using hybridomas[30–31]. Hybridomas are the product of the fusion of B-lymphocytes with certain myeloma cell lines. The fused cells are capable of secreting, in culture, large amounts of homologous antibody of the specificity determined by the original B-lymphocyte. In theory it should be possible to select the specificity of the antibody produced in this manner by characterizing the surface immunoglobulins of the B-lymphocytes used. It could be possible to detect the right B-lymphocytes by making use of the unique properties of anti-idiotype antisera to react with the antigen-combining site of the surface immunoglobulins enabling separation of B-lymphocytes with the correct specificity.

Acknowledgement

I would like to thank Dr D. Anstee for his many helpful discussions and continuous encouragement.

References

1. Frangione, B., Franklin, E. C., Fudenberg, H. H. and Koshland, M. E. (1966). Structural studies of human γ G-myeloma proteins of different antigenic subgroups and genetic specificities. *J. Exp. Med.*, **124**, 715
2. Wang, A. C. and Fudenberg, H. H. (1969). Genetic control of gamma chain synthesis: A chemical and evolutionary study of the Gm(a) factor of immunoglobulins. *J. Molec. Biol.*, **45**, 493
3. Milstein, C. P., Syeinberg, A. G., McLaughlin, C. I. and Solomon, A. (1974). Amino-acid sequence change associated with genetic marker Inv (2) of human immunoglobulin. *Nature*, **248**, 160
4. Devey, M. E. and Voak, D. (1974). A critical study of the IgG subclasses of Rh anti-D antibodies formed in pregnancy and in immunized volunteers. *Immunology*, **27**, 1073
5. Vaughan, J. H., Barnett, E. V. and Leddy, J. P. (1966). Autosensitivity diseases. Immunologic and pathogenetic concepts in lupus erythematosus, rheumatoid arthritis and haemolytic anaemia. *New Engl. J. Med.*, **275**, 1426
6. Grubb, R. (1956). Agglutination of erythrocytes coated with 'incomplete' anti-Rh by certain rheumatoid arthritic sera and some other sera. The existence of human serum groups. *Acta Path. Microbiol. Scand.*, **39**, 195
7. Review of the notation for the allotypic and related markers of human immunoglobulins (1976). *J. Immunogenet.*, **3**, 357
8. Leikola, J. (1975). Transfusion reactions caused by IgA and other plasma proteins. *Special symposium held at the XIV Congress of the International Society of Blood Transfusion*, Helsinki
9. Konugres, A. A., Holbrook, E. R. and Corcoran, P. A. (1966). Another source of error in red cell typing. *Transfusion*, **6**, 80

10. Litwin, S. D. (1973). Allotype preference in human Rh antibodies. *J. Immunol.*, **110**, 717
11. Pineda, A. A. and Taswell, H. F. (1975). Transfusion reactions associated with anti-IgA antibodies: Report of four cases and review of the literature. *Transfusion*, **15**, 10
12. Leikola, J., Koistinen, J., Lehtinen, M. and Virolainen, M. (1973). IgA-induced anaphylactic transfusion reactions: A report of four cases. *Blood*, **42**, 111
13. Miller, W. V., Holland, P. V., Sugarbaker, E., Strober, W. and Waldmann, T. A. (1970). Anaphylactic reactions to IgA: A difficult transfusion problem. *Am. J. Clin. Path.*, **54**, 618
14. Vyas, G. N., Perkins, H. A. and Fudenberg, H. H. (1968). Anaphylactoid transfusion reaction associated with anti-IgA. *Lancet*, **ii**, 312
15. Vyas, G. N. and Fudenberg, H. H. (1970). Immunobiology of human anti-IgA: A serologic and immunogenetic study of immunisation to IgA in transfusion and pregnancy. *Clin. Genet.*, **1**, 45
16. Koistinen, J. and Leikola, J. (1977). Weak anti-IgA antibodies with limited specificity and non-haemolytic transfusion reactions. *Vox. Sang.*, **32**, 77
17. Rivat, L., Rivat, C., Daveau, M. and Ropartz, C. (1977). Comparative frequencies of anti-IgA antibodies among patients with anaphylactic transfusion reactions and among normal blood donors. *Clin. Immunol. Immunopathol.*, **7**, 340
18. Johansson, S. G. O., Högman, C. F. and Killander, J. (1968). Quantitative immunoglobulin determination. Comparison of two methods. Estimation of normal levels and levels in persons lacking IgA or IgD. *Acta Path. Microbiol. Scand.*, **74**, 519
19. Natvig, J. B., Harboe, M., Fausa, O. and Tveit, A. (1971). Family studies in individuals with selective absence of γA-globulin. *Clin. Exp. Immunol.*, **8**, 229
20. Frommel, D., Moullec, J., Lambin, P. and Fine, J. M. (1973). Selective serum IgA deficiency. Frequency among 15 200 French blood donors. *Vox Sang.*, **25**, 513
21. Koistinen, J. (1975). Selective IgA deficiency in blood donors. *Vox. Sang.*, **29**, 192
22. Vyas, G. N., Perkins, H. A., Yang, Y–M. and Basantani, G. K. (1975). Healthy blood donors with selective absence of immunoglobulin A: prevention of anaphylactic transfusion reactions caused by antibodies to IgA. *J. Lab. Clin. Med.*, **85**, 838
23. Holt, P. D. J., Tandy, N. P. and Anstee, D. J. (1977). Screening of blood donors for IgA deficiency: a study of the donor population of south-west England. *J. Clin. Path.*, **30**, 1007
24. Lawton, A. R., Royal, S. A., Self, K. S. and Cooper, M. D. (1972). IgA determinations on B-lymphocytes in patients with deficiency of circulating IgA. *J. Lab. Clin. Med.*, **80**, 26
25. Deutsch, H. F. and MacKenzie, M. R. (1964). Serological demonstration of antigenic heterogeneity of individual human γ₁-macroglobulins. *Nature*, **201**, 87
26. Franklin, E. C. and Frangione, B. (1967). Two serologically distinguishable subclasses of μ-chains of human macroglobulins. *J. Immunol.*, **99**, 810
27. Wells, J. V., Bleumers, J. F. and Fudenberg, H. H. (1973). Human anti-IgM iso-antibodies: detection of IgM allotypic markers. *Proc. Nat. Acad. Sci.*, **70**, 827

28. Leikola, J., Fudenberg, H. H., Vyas, G. N. and Perkins, H. A. (1971). Isoanti-
bodies to human IgM: serologic and immunochemical investigations. *J. Immunol.*,
106, 1147
29. Natvig, J. B., Kunkel, H. G. and Joslim, F. G. (1969). Delineation of two
antigenic markers "non-a" and "non-g" related to the genetic antigens of human
globulin. *J. Immunol.*, **102,** 611
30. Kohler, G. and Milstein, C. (1975). Continuous cultures of fused cells secreting
antibody of predefined specificity. *Nature*, **256,** 495
31. Pearson, T., Galfre, G., Zeigler, A. and Milstein, C. (1977). A myeloma hybrid
producing antibody specific for an allotypic determinant on 'IgD-like' molecules
of the mouse. *Eur. J. Immunol.*, **7,** 684

10

Monoclonal proteins
J. Kohn

10.1 INTRODUCTION   115

10.2 NOMENCLATURE   116

10.3 AETIOLOGY   116

10.4 INCIDENCE   117

10.5 LABORATORY INVESTIGATION OF SERUM PROTEINS   119
     10.5.1 *Artefacts on serum electrophoresis*   121
     10.5.2 *Multiple paraproteins*   122
     10.5.3 *Transient paraproteins*   122
     10.5.4 *Cryoglobulins*   123
     10.5.5 *Myeloma without a paraprotein*   123

10.6 LABORATORY INVESTIGATION OF URINE   123

10.7 MACROGLOBULINAEMIA   124

10.8 BENIGN PARAPROTEINAEMIA   124

     10.8.1 *Criteria of benign paraproteinaemia*   126

10.1 INTRODUCTION

I should like to discuss the implications and the approach to dealing with those cases in which the serum contains a monoclonal band. They frequently cause a flurry and flutter in every laboratory the moment they are seen and start off a chain of activities which is sometimes purposeful and provides the information that is wanted, but which not infrequently leads to more mysteries.

A monoclonal protein is synthesized by one clone of cells; and therefore the molecules have the same charge, the same size, and the same shape. They will behave in a similar way in an electric field, and will be characterized by a discrete band, which on zone electrophoresis has very clearly defined sharp edges, in contrast to the polyclonal increase of gammaglobulins which is more blurred. This is a very important point, as the distinction between a polyclonal and a monoclonal protein is not always easy to make. A number of procedures which are used to investigate paraproteins may influence their appearance. A typical example would be the use of an instrument which gives too short a separation. The gamma region is either squeezed to the degree where it looks like a paraprotein or is so dense that one cannot see a paraprotein which might be present.

Paraproteins are immunoglobulins and would therefore be expected to have antibody characteristics. It is very likely that in fact they are antibodies and in a number of instances antibody activity has been demonstrated, e.g. antistreptolysin, anti-rheumatoid factor, anti-myelin, etc. However in the overwhelming majority of cases the paraproteins are antibodies still in search of their corresponding antigens. Commonly these monoclonal proteins are of autoimmune antibody type. In view of the enormous numbers of possible substances acting as antigen this is not surprising.

10.2   NOMENCLATURE

Many names have been proposed for these proteins, particularly for the benign forms. Paraprotein is my personal choice. It is an easy word and it can be permutated, e.g. paraproteinaemia – and used in other combinations. It is perfectly simple to qualify what one means by it.

10.3   AETIOLOGY

The monoclonal immunoglobulins are found in a number of conditions which can be divided roughly into the following classes:–
   multiple myeloma
   Waldenström's macroglobinaemia
   heavy chain diseases
   light chain diseases
   lichen myxoedematosis (papular mucinosis)
   malignant lymphomas
   amyloidosis
   monocytic leukaemias

The incidence of paraprotein class follows the incidence of the normal immunoglobulins. That means that IgG is commonest, then IgA, IgM, IgD, and IgE. A separate group are the Bence Jones or the light-chain paraprotein-aemias (Table 10.1).

Monoclonal proteins in the serum can also occur without association with any recognized pathology. These have been classified as idiopathic or benign, and their aetiology and pathogenesis still remain obscure. There is very little known about them except that certain factors are associated with their presence. These include age, a genetic disposition – (on a number of occasions there have been recorded familial occurrences of monoclonal proteins); they are also much more common in immune deficiency states. Certain correlations of paraproteins with diseases are well-known, but not necessarily proven as a causative association.

Although a relationship between cancer and the occurrence of paraproteins has been reported by several authors it is still no more than a hypothesis. Many workers tend to agree that the incidence of paraproteinaemia in cancer is not greater than that expected in a corresponding age group.

The range of concentration of paraprotein is wide. The levels can vary from about 0.1 g/l to 100 g/l and even more. It must be remembered that when the paraproteins become manifest in a disease like a myeloma, it has taken a very long time before they have been detected. In the case of IgA, for instance, it may take 17–21 years before sufficient paraprotein is being synthesized to be detectable in the serum, and for IgG the time factor is even longer. There is, therefore, an extremely long symptomless period. The doubling time has been estimated at something in the region of 6.3 months.

One can assume that the tumour mass is reflected in the amount of para-protein present, provided allowances are made for the turnover rate. The most important application of the assessment of the amount of paraprotein is in the management of disease and to some extent in the differential diagnosis between benign or malignant conditions.

10.4 INCIDENCE

The incidence of paraproteinaemia depends on age. In a normal healthy population one can expect something of the order of 0.2% below the age of 60; i.e. 2 out of every 1000 will produce a paraprotein in their blood, usually completely unsuspected.

In collaboration with the South London Blood Transfusion Centre we investigated 9420 blood donors for the presence of monoclonal bands, and of these 19 had a definite paraproteinaemia. In 18 cases it was of the IgG

TABLE 10.1 Incidence of paraproteinaemia in aged populations

Author	Age group	Population group	No. examined	Incidence Paraproteinaemia	Incidence Overt myeloma
Fine et al.	>68	Old people's home	500	3.0%	0.4%
Hallen	>50	Old people's home	294	3.1%	0.0%
Axelsson et al.	>70	General population	3674	1.6%	0.3%
Walsh et al.	>50	Psychiatric hospital	1011	2.1%	0.5%
Kohn et al.	>60	Outpatients geriatric	806	1.8%	1.2%
Kohn et al.	>60	Inpatients geriatric	1000	3.2%	2.6%
Englisowa et al.	65–79		369	1.6%	
	80–90		51	11.7%	?
	>90		26	19.0%	
Radl et al. (unpublished)	>95	Old people's home	73	19.0%	?
Zawadzki	>70	Inpatients	748	7.5%	2.0%

type and in one case an IgM. Similar results were obtained in many other studies all over the world. One can therefore expect that in the normal population at large, there will be about that amount of symptomless – let us call it benign – paraproteinaemia. Our donors with paraproteinaemia have been followed up, some of them for as long as 10 years, and in only one case is there a slight suspicion that there may be something wrong with the donor but he is still completely symptomless. So far, the paraproteinaemia in our donors can be regarded as benign. I must repeat that this is a population at large, and not in patients who come to the outpatient clinic or are admitted to hospital.

The incidence increase very dramatically with age and by the time people reach 90 and over – and there are Russian and Dutch data available – the incidence of cases of paraproteinaemia becomes something of the order of 17–19%. It appears that if one lived long enough, say to a ripe age of 120, then everybody would have a paraproteinaemia. During the course of a lifetime one is exposed to so many antigenic insults that one day a plasma cell will say that enough is enough and will start to proliferate in a benign or a malignant fashion.

10.5 LABORATORY INVESTIGATION OF SERUM PROTEINS

How do we proceed with the investigation of paraproteinaemia? If one sticks to a certain investigation pattern, one should not encounter major problems (see Tables 10.2 and 10.3).

The total protein should be estimated although this is not particularly useful. Serum electrophoresis will show whether or not there is a paraprotein (a monoclonal band) present; this must be sharply defined, and clearly outlined. The band must be quantitated, preferably by scanning or elution. This is most important for the management of disease, for serial estimations are used to assess the response to treatment. If scanning is used it is possible to separate visually the paraprotein component of the peak from the underlying immunoglobulin background. This can then be measured by planimetry or weighing and a more accurate estimation obtained.

An immunoglobulin estimation must be performed. It is important to stress that it should be performed only for the non-committed immunoglobulins but not for the paraprotein. Immunochemical paraprotein estimation is very unreliable although unfortunately it is carried out in laboratories all over the world (Table 10.4). Three cases are shown. One case of IgG myeloma, one of IgA and one of IgM. They have been quantitated by commercially available immunoplates. There is nothing wrong with the immunoplates as such, but there are large differences in the results and they are hardly worth the paper that they are written on. Moreover, they are grossly misleading. If a patient is followed up, perhaps starting with something that has, say, a low result, and then using the next batch of a different antiserum which gives a high result, one might be led to think that the patient's condition is deteriorating, and vice versa.

Table 10.2   Laboratory investigations of serum proteins

1. Total protein
2. Serum electrophoresis
3. Estimation of paraprotein, e.g. scanning
4. Immunoelectrophoresis or immunofixation
5. Immunoglobulin quantitation
6. Light chain typing

   Note: Ideally blood should be collected and serum separated at 37 °C.
   No anticoagulants

Table 10.3   Urine investigations: absolutely essential

1. Urine electrophoresis for presence of Bence Jones protein (monoclonal light chains)
2. Quantitation of Bence Jones protein (very helpful in assessment and follow-up)

   Note: Albustix may not react with Bence Jones protein. The boiling test is not reliable.
   If urine is not concentrated B.J protein can be missed in about 40% of cases on
   electrophoresis

Table 10.4   Paraproteins from three cases of immunocytoma quantitated by commercial immunodiffusion plates

	Commercial immunodiffusion plates					
	1	2	3	4	5	6
IgG myeloma	640	1190	780	960	0450	895
IgA myeloma	660	516	1060	1560	448	660
IgM paraprotein	370	500	513	300	418	392

Values in mg/dl

The next step is immunoelectrophoresis is order to try to classify and to type the paraprotein. Immunofixation can also be used for this purpose. The light-chain typing should be performed in all cases. There are indications that certain light-chain types carry a less favourable prognosis. Here arises a question that I have heard many times and that has some validity: is it important to know whether or not there is an IgG-K, or an IgG sub-type, 1, 2, 3 or 4? It is a pertinent question and one that is difficult to answer. There is, however, a good answer if a distinction has to be drawn between an IgG or an IgA myeloma and an IgM. Their treatment is different. There are also some prognostic indications to be gained.

10.5.1 Artefacts on serum electrophoresis

What can simulate a monoclonal protein? 'Zoning' is one of the most common – a fine banding often seen in the gamma region. Fibrinogen is a homogeneous protein which may cause interpretation problems. Haemoglobin, if present, may produce an appearance of monoclonicity. Transferrin may simulate a paraprotein, particularly when there is an immunodeficiency present. Lysozyme will produce a very slow discrete band beyond the gamma region. Raised C-reactive protein may produce a fine band in the mid-gamma region. Then there may be immunoglobulin aggregation, e.g. in uraemia. A very common phenomenon is particulate material sticking on the application line. (The obvious solution is to make sure that the serum sample is well spun or filtered through a suitable membrane).

Cryoglobulins may present a problem. Cryoglobulins are globulins that precipitate at low temperature, and sometimes even at room temperature. If the blood is collected in a cold syringe or, what is more important, if it is left to separate out in the cold, or even at room temperature, then cryoglobulins may precipitate; one will find them in the clot, and there will be none left in the serum. This is not all that uncommon and it usually applies to the IgM type of cryoparaproteins, although it may also happen with others.

Denaturation is not uncommon. Bacterial contamination, if a specimen is left standing for prolonged periods of time, may play a very serious role. IgG$_3$ seems to be particularly prone to denaturation. Then come the more difficult and less obvious problems when the paraprotein band is difficult to demonstrate because it is hidden under large and heavily stained fractions, for instance under the beta, less often the alpha fraction. The Bence Jones protein in the serum, the light chain on its own, a small and usually weak band, is often missed if the electrophoretic separation is not sufficiently sharp. The alpha heavy-chain disease paraprotein, i.e. the heavy chain on its own, is not the discrete band usually seen in other types of monoclonal proteins, it is rather fuzzy and broad.

IgD paraproteins are unstable, migrating at different speeds after varying periods of storage. It may be first seen in the gamma region, and subsequently be found in the alpha region. The IgD bands are not clear cut and have often been missed. IgD is sometimes confused with Bence Jones or light-chain paraproteinaemia as they display similar characteristics, i.e. a very marked immunosuppression and frequently relatively low total protein values.

10.5.2   Multiple paraproteins

Multiple discrete bands in the gamma region on electrophoresis are not an uncommon phenomenon. We have collected over a hundred cases in our Protein Unit. The name of multiclonicity is the exception rather than the rule, and we would suggest the term multiband paraprotein which does not prejudge the nature of the bands.

The multiband pattern can be the result of polymerization, which is quite common, particularly with IgA with the paraproteins in a dimer or even tetramer form or complexing with albumin for instance. Enzymatic immunoglobulin breakdown is not uncommon and has been seen to happen even in the patient's circulation, e.g. in burns. On the 5th or 6th day after a burn a pattern is seen sometimes which is indistinguishable from that seen after papain digestion. Probably the most common multiband paraproteinaemia is a combination of a paraprotein with a Bence Jones protein in the serum. Another example is a tribe of clones – a number of related clones producing bands at the same time. This has been observed in marrow transplant patients which start to produce immunoglobulins, but only some clones will respond initially. There is thus a progressive appearance of multiple bands as the graft 'takes' until they fuse to produce the diffuse gamma region.

Finally, much less common the genuine, multiclonal paraproteinaemias. The clinical correlation of the multiband paraproteinaemias does not seem to differ from that of monoclonal ones.

10.5.3   Transient paraproteins

The so-called transient paraproteins are yet another type of monoclonal protein. They are very often – or so we think – produced by antigenic stimulation. The typical pattern is of the monoclonal peak appearing and then disappearing within a matter of weeks. They are most often to be found in young children, sometimes in connection with immunodeficiencies.

10.5.4   Cryoglobulins

I have already said that the problem with cryoglobulins lies in the method of collecting the specimens. IgM are the most common but frequently so-called mixed cryoglobulins will be found. We have even seen a few cases of cryo-Bence Jones in which the urine gelled very nicely even at room temperature.

The other group, very rare, which we have seen among blood donors whom we have investigated, are the pyroglobulins; these precipitate at the temperature used for the inactivation of complement. They too may be paraproteins.

10.5.5   Myeloma without a paraprotein

There is a further problem – the failure to demonstrate a monoclonal protein in clinically proven cases of myeloma. This may be due to the fact that they are just not there. It may be one of the very rare immunocytomas which do not excrete or synthesize paraproteins, called by some authors the non-excreting or non-secreting myeloma.

10.6   LABORATORY INVESTIGATION OF URINE

Monoclonal free light chains – Bence Jones protein – may be present in the urine in about 65% of myelomas. Heterogeneous or polyclonal free light chains may be present in situations of renal tubular damage or hyper-stimulation of the immune system. Normal plasma cells produce traces of free light chains in excess. These are usually largely reabsorbed in the renal tubule, about 40 mg/day appearing in the urine in normal people.

Concentrated (up to 300 times) and unconcentrated urine should be electrophoresed alongside a diluted sample of the same patient's serum. Where mobilities of the paraprotein band in the serum are the same as in the urine it is very likely that the paraprotein is leaking through a damaged kidney. Where, however, there is only a monoclonal band in the urine without the albumin band present, then a Bence Jones protein is the most likely diagnosis. Identification must be performed by immunochemical means. The most common pitfalls, again, are the presence of haemoglobin, transferrin, Ig fragments, Lysozyme (which is a very slow one), and leaking paraproteins which will produce a monoclonal band in the urine. There are cases in which Bence Jones protein is only present in the serum in a tetrameric form, with a molecular weight of about 88 000 daltons. Then it is not found in the urine.

The Bence Jones myeloma is perhaps the most commonly missed. The ESR in a Bence Jones type myeloma is usually low, whereas it is high in the other types of myeloma. Immunosuppression is a very common feature. This combined with a low total protein and normal ESR should draw attention to the possible presence of a Bence Jones myeloma.

10.7   MACROGLOBULINAEMIA

Macroglobulinaemia is a condition in which there is an IgM paraprotein in the serum associated with a low grade malignant lymphoma. One form carries the name of Waldenström and should not be confused with the second Waldenström's disease – purpura-hypergammaglobulinaemia which represents polyclonal high molecular weight IgG complexes and which is usually benign.

It was recently noticed that peripheral neuropathies are occasionally associated with IgM paraproteins; some of these have been shown to be anti-myelin antibodies.

Some of the problems of identification have been mentioned. One not-too-well known fact is that PEG 6000 at about 8% precipitates IgM paraproteins. It does not precipitate IgA and only partially IgG; this method can be used for differentiation purposes if more sophisticated laboratory facilities are not available. Clinically the importance of IgM paraproteinaemia lies in the risk of hyperviscosity. The treatment is different from that of the other paraproteinaemias.

10.8   BENIGN PARAPROTEINAEMIA (Table 10.5)

This group poses a very difficult problem. The incidence depends primarily on the population studied. One could adopt a very simple rule of thumb that in the population at large paraproteins present are regarded as non-malignant unless proved otherwise. However in hospital patients with symptoms, a paraproteinaemia is malignant unless proved to be benign and it must be followed up for at least 5 years before it can be called benign. They are mostly IgG or IgM (Table 10.2). Benign IgA paraproteinaemias, particularly of the lambda type, must be rare.

In the first 1000 geriatric patients in a Sheffield hospital screened for the presence of paraproteinaemia we found 30 patients with paraproteinaemia and of those 24 were malignant, typical myelomas. They went undetected probably because the patients were old people with a variety of symptoms. In these cases it may be justifiable to talk about a senile myeloma which would be relatively 'symptom poor' – as the Germans would say.

What is the possible aetiology of the benign paraproteinaemias? Unfortunately there are no biochemical or structural differences, no class or sub-class differences and there is no difference in the electron microscope findings. There may be two types of paraproteinaemia just as the adenoma is benign and the carcinoma is malignant. It may be a committed clone, which has not been stimulated. It may be that by feedback inhibition the proliferation is kept in check. It may be malignant from the beginning but with the brake on – probably an immunological one. Otherwise it is extremely difficult to explain a stable level of paraprotein for a long time without an underlying mechanism keeping the synthesis in check.

TABLE 10.5 Criteria of benign paraproteinaemia

1. No clinical symptoms related to myeloma or macroglobulinaemia
2. No palpable enlargement of lymph nodes, spleen or liver
3. Negative X-ray
4. Negative bone marrow
5. Amount of abnormal protein usually <10 g/l (over 20 g/l only in 10% of cases)
6. Bence Jones in urine absent.
7. Follow-up at least 5 years without evidence of malignancy

TABLE 10.6 Criteria of malignancy

1. Characteristic bone marrow findings
2. X-ray findings:–
   (a) Discrete osteolytic lesions
   (b) Diffuse osteoporosis with collapsed vertebrae or pathological fractures without obvious cause
3. Amounts of paraprotein estimated by scanning or elution of electrophoretic pattern exceeding:–
   20 g/l in cases of IgG paraproteinaemia
   10 g/l in cases of IgA paraproteinaemia
   10 g/l in cases of IgM paraproteinaemia
   are suggestive of malignancy
4. IgD and IgE paraproteinaemia are invariably malignant.
5. Significant amounts of Bence Jones protein (free light chains) exceeding 1 g/l almost invariably indicate a malignant condition
6. Progressive increase of paraprotein levels
7. Immunosuppression of 'non-committed' immunoglobulins

10.8.1   Criteria of benign paraproteinaemia

These are shown in Table 10.5.

From the point of view of the protein laboratory the distinction between benign and malignant is one of the most important problems. The more relevant clinical information that can be obtained, the more likely is the laboratory to provide the clinician with relevant data helpful in the management of the case.

References

1. Axelsson, U., Bachman, R. and Hallen, J. (1966). Frequency of pathological proteins (M components) in 6,995 sera from an adult population. *Acta Med. Scand.,* **179**, 235
2. Englisowa, M., Englis, M., Kyral, V., Kourilek, K. and Drovak, K. (1968). Changes of immunoglobulin synthesis in old people. *Exp. Gerontol.,* **3**, 125
3. Fine, J. M., Derycke, C. and Boffa, G. A. (1966). Les formes atypiques et essentialles de dysglobulinémies. *Rev. Méd. Tours,* **2**, 193
4. Hallen, J. (1963). Frequency of abnormal serum globulins (M components) in the aged. *Acta. Med. Scand.,* **173**, 737
5. Kohn, J. and Srivastava, P. C. (1972). Paraproteins in Blood donors and the aged, benign and malignant. *Prot. Biol. Fluids,* **20**, 257
6. Walsh, N. P., McSweeney, J. R. and Russell, M. P. (1971). Paraprotein screening in a psychiatric hospital. *J. Irish Med. Assoc.,* **64**, 12
7. Zawadzki, Z. A. and Edwards, G. A. (1972). Nonmyelomatous monoclonal immunoglobulinaemia. *Progr. Clin. Immunol.,* **1**, 105

11

Iron binding proteins
A. Jacobs

11.1	INTRODUCTION	127
11.2	IRON METABOLISM	128
	11.2.1 *Ferritin and transferrin synthesis*	129
11.3	TRANSFERRIN	129
	11.3.1 *Clinical value of transferrin measurements*	129
	11.3.2 *Kinetic measurements of iron turnover*	130
11.4	FERRITIN	132
	11.4.1 *Clinical value of ferritin measurements*	132
	11.4.2 *Other variations in serum ferritin levels*	132
11.5	CONCLUSIONS	133

11.1 INTRODUCTION

Iron is a highly reactive metal which will bind to a wide variety of biological substances including sugars, amino acids, nucleotides, peptides and proteins. To discuss iron binding proteins is to discuss almost all human proteins. In this paper I intend to discuss the role of the specific iron binding proteins, transferrin and ferritin, in relation to the physiology and pathology of iron transport and metabolism.

Because iron is so highly reactive, it is also extremely toxic; by binding to proteins and enzymes it can interfere with many metabolic reactions. During the course of evolution the body has devised specific proteins which play a major role in iron metabolism and which ensure that storage and transport are free from toxic effects. The principal storage protein, ferritin, is phylogenetically even more ancient than the immunoglobulins, being found in all animal species and in all plant species down to the fungi.

11.2   IRON METABOLISM

The main metabolic pathways for iron in the human body are summarized in Figure 11.1 Plasma iron, or transferrin iron, occupies a central position with regard to iron metabolism. Most of the iron passing from one site to another passes through this plasma pool. The major portion of the plasma iron is destined for bone marrow erythrocytes. Iron is taken up from transferrin by the red cell precursors where it is processed into haemoglobin. Mature red cells are released into the circulation where they remain for 100–110 days and then end their life-span by being taken up by the reticuloendothelial system. Haemoglobulin is digested, the haeme ring cleaved, and iron mobilized to be recycled back to the plasma. There is also a limited amount of ineffective erythropoiesis where iron is incorporated into haemoglobin but the red cells do not survive and their iron is recycled within the marrow cavity. Iron also passes to non-erythroid tissues because most cells have an iron requirement for myoglobin or for iron containing enzymes.

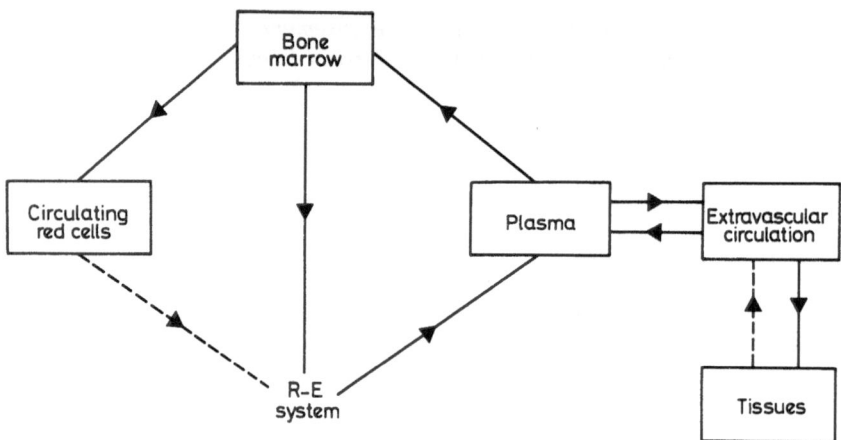

Figure 11.1   Schematic diagram of the major iron metabolic pathways

11.2.1   Ferritin and transferrin synthesis

Ferritin is the iron storage protein present in the RE cells and the iron storage organs, but almost all cells have the capability to synthesize ferritin. Transferrin is synthesized largely in the liver.

The synthesis of both these proteins is controlled by the iron supply. Ferritin synthesis is stimulated by increased iron supply at the cellular level, whilst transferrin synthesis is inhibited.

11.3   TRANSFERRIN

Transferrin is a β-globulin of molecular weight 75 000–80 000 daltons consisting of a single polypeptide chain. The primary structure of the molecule has not been completely defined but it would appear that there has been reduplication of the molecule during evolution.

Each transferrin molecule binds two atoms of ferric iron; the iron binding sites are believed to consist of three tyrosine residues together with two other residues, the iron atom being associated with a carbonate or bicarbonate anion. There remains considerable debate as to the functional equivalence of the two iron binding sites on the molecule, and the mechanism of binding and release is unknown. *In vitro* evidence has shown, however, that the binding becomes progressively looser as the pH falls until the bond dissociates completely at pH 4.5. The critical factor in binding iron to the transferrin molecule would appear to be the anion. Carbonate can be replaced by citrate, malate or oxalate. Binding with oxalate, however, creates a non-reversible bonding. The current hypothesis is that in the release of iron from transferrin, the anion is released first rendering the iron molecule more loosely bound.

Red-cell precursors have specific transferrin receptors on the cell surface which bind transferrin, accept the released iron and then allow the transferrin to recirculate.

11.3.1   Clinical value of transferrin measurements

Transferrin is usually measured as total iron binding capacity (TIBC) because the haematologist is primarily interested in actual and potential iron transport rather than the protein itself. The measurement of serum iron allows the calculation of the transferrin saturation, usually about 30% in the normal individual.

In *iron deficiency* there is increased transferrin synthesis, increased TIBC, low serum iron and low transferrin saturation. In *infections* and *chronic inflammation* there is decreased transferrin synthesis, low TIBC, low serum iron and a low saturation. Neither low serum iron nor a low saturation are diagnostic of iron deficiency. In *iron overload* transferrin saturation approaches 100% but this is of doubtful clinical value.

Serum iron determinations are of very limited value to the haematologist because of the extreme variability of serum levels within the individual. There is marked, and often variable, diurnal variation, maximal levels being found in early morning. Even with samples taken at the same time each day, day-to-day variations in the normal individual may fluctuate from apparent deficiency to apparent overload.

Although subject to enormous variation and misinterpretation, serum iron and TIBC has been used to differentiate patients who have a normal but "low" haemoglobin concentration from those truly anaemic due to iron deficiency.

11.3.2 Kinetic measurements of iron turnover

A more useful aspect of transferrin in clinical diagnosis lies in the kinetics of iron transport. The main interest is in bone marrow erythroid function and

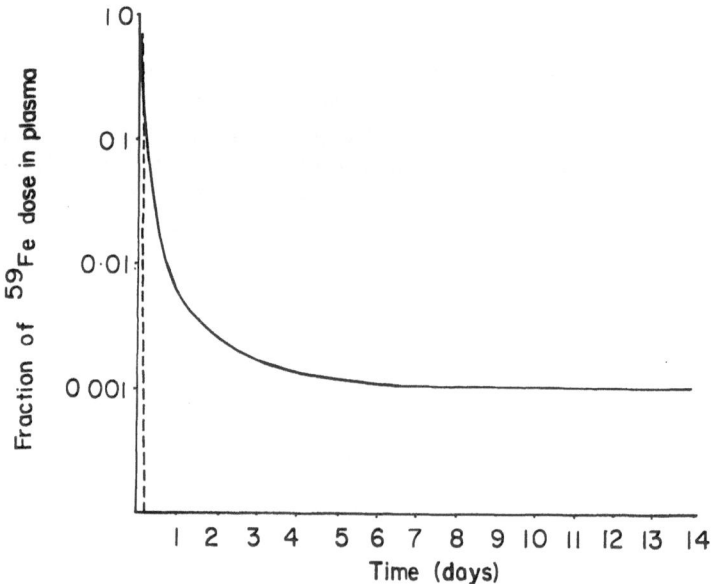

Figure 11.2 ^{59}Fe transferrin clearance in the normal individual

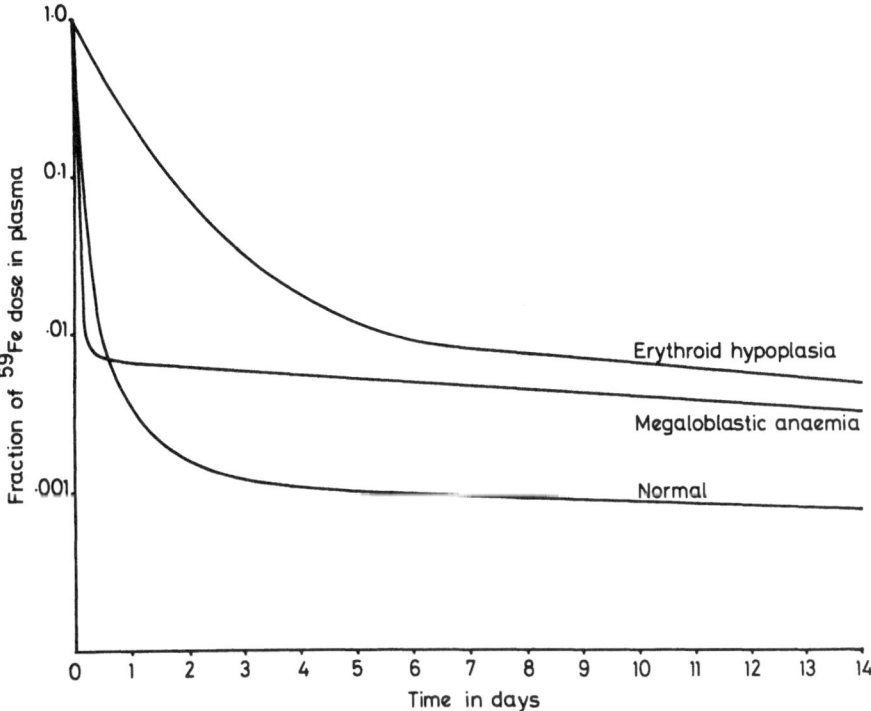

Figure 11.3 ^{59}Fe transferrin clearance in pathological erythropoietic states

the relative efficiency of the bone marrow. As most of the iron travelling on transferrin is destined for erythropoiesis, a measurement of rate of disappearance of iron can give an indication of erythroid function. The clearance of ^{59}Fe labelled transferrin in normal subjects is shown in Figure 11.2. The clearance of labelled transferrin under different physiological conditions of erythropoiesis is shown in Figure 11.3. In megaloblastic erythropoiesis there is increased bone marrow activity and increased initial utilization of iron. Increased red cell destruction and the steady state is set at a higher level than in the normal. In erythroid hypoplasia initial clearance is reduced and there is further increase in feedback to the serum.

By analysis of the clearance curves it is possible to calculate the total marrow iron turnover (MIT). As the total red cell iron within the body is known as is the amount of iron contained within each red cell, it is possible to calculate the mean red cell production – about 2 million cells per second – and the red cell life-span. This provides an alternative technique to iron labelling.

11.4 FERRITIN

Whilst it has been known for many years that transferrin is the circulating iron transport protein, it has always been assumed that ferritin was a storage protein that only existed within cells. It is now known that significant quantities of ferritin leak from or are secreted by cells and can be found in the serum.

The ferritin molecule is a large, electron dense molecule consisting of a protein shell 120 angstrom units in diameter enclosing an iron core of 72–75 angstrom units in diameter and a molecular weight between 0.5 and 1.0 million daltons. A model of the ferritin molecule has recently been described by Harrison (1977). Iron enters the molecule in the ferrous form and is deposited as ferric iron crystals, the inner core having a potential capacity of about 4000 atoms. Mobilization of iron from the ferritin molecule requires the iron to be converted from the ferric to ferrous form but the precise mechanisms of uptake and release have not been clearly defined.

Serum ferritin levels have been shown to correlate well with stainable iron in bone marrow aspirates, and data from patients with iron overload show that this correlation holds also for extramedullary iron stores.

11.4.1 Clinical value of ferritin measurements

In the normal population serum ferritin levels show a skewed distribution with higher levels in males than in females. In males the range is from about 10–400 μg/l with a mean of 123 μg/l, and in females about 10–200 μg/l with a mean of 56 μg/l. At these levels 1 μg/l of serum ferritin appears to be equivalent to 8 mg of storage iron and these values for serum ferritin can be converted into total body storage iron, about 1000 mg for males and 450 mg for females.

Serum ferritin estimation can, therefore, be used as a measurement of total body iron stores and can be used to monitor response to treatment.

Serum ferritin levels are low in iron deficiency anaemia and rise on treatment with ferrous sulphate. Treatment may be continued until the iron stores have attained normal levels.

Serum ferritin levels are grossly raised in iron overload and the effectiveness of chelation therapy can be monitored by the reduction in ferritin levels. Similar possibilities are available for monitoring the effectiveness of repeated phlebotomy in the treatment of idiopathic haemochromatosis.

11.4.2 Other variations in serum ferritin levels

Serum ferritin concentrations are stable in the normal individual and free from diurnal variation seen in transferrin levels.

Ferritin is an acute phase reactant protein, levels rising after an acute insult. Ferritin levels rise markedly in the 3 days following myocardial infarction, levels rising as the serum iron and transferrin fall. A similar change may be seen in the postoperative period, maximal levels being reached 2–3 days after surgery.

Serum ferritin levels are increased in acute infections, trauma and any chronic inflammatory condition. Very high levels are seen in liver cell damage, either acute hepatitis or alcoholic liver damage.

Serum ferritin is also increased in acute leukaemia.

11.5 CONCLUSIONS

Although it is possible to measure serum iron, transferrin and ferritin, there is no such thing as a test for iron deficiency or iron overload.

Transport iron can be measured but one must remain aware of the tremendous diurnal and individual variation. The results will only show the amount of iron in the transport phase at that point in time.

Storage iron can be measured as serum ferritin, and, in the absence of confusing factors, this is an excellent test but it will tell you nothing about the patient except the amount of storage iron present.

Bibliography

Jacobs, A. and Worwood, M. (eds.) *Iron in Biochemistry and Medicine*. (New York: Academic Press)

Harrison, P. M. (1977). Ferritin; iron storage molecule. *Sem. Haematol.*, **14**, 55

Jacobs, A. (1977). Disorders of iron metabolism. In: Hoffbrand *et al.* (eds.) *Recent Advances in Haematology II*. (Edinburgh and London: Churchill Livingstone)

Cavill, I., Ricketts, C. and Jacobs, A. (1977). *Clin. Haematol.*, **6**, 583

Jacobs, A. and Worwood, M. (1975). The biochemistry of ferritin and its clinical implications. *Progress in Haemotology 9*. (New York: Grune and Stratton)

12

Albumin
Linda Smith

12.1 THE CLINICAL VALUE OF SERUM ALBUMIN
    MEASUREMENT   136
    12.1.1 *Malnutrition and malabsorption*   136
    12.1.2 *Protein-losing states*   136
    12.1.3 *Liver disease*   137
    12.1.4 *Malignancy*   137
12.2 STANDARDIZATION OF SERUM ALBUMIN
    MEASUREMENT   137
    12.2.1 *Purity of various albumin preparations*   138
        12.2.1.1 *The relationship between dry weight and*
                  albumin concentration   138
        12.2.1.2 *The presence of protein impurities in the*
                  products   138
    12.2.2 *The behaviour of various albumin preparations in the*
            estimation of albumin and total protein   140
        12.2.2.1 *The biuret reaction for total protein*
                  measurement   149
        12.2.2.2 *Bromocreso green dye binding (BCG)*   140
        12.2.2.3 *Rocket-immunoelectrophoresis (RIEP)*
                  and the automated immunoprecipitin   140
                  (AIP) techniques
    12.2.3 *The choice of a suitable preparation for use as a standard* 141

12.3   PROBLEMS WITH ALBUMIN ANALYSIS   142
       12.3.1   Chemical methods   142
       12.3.2   Immunochemical methods   143
                12.3.2.1   Method comparison   143

12.4   THE CHOICE OF METHOD FOR ALBUMIN ANALYSIS   145

12.5   PROBLEMS ASSOCIATED WITH CHANGING TO
       IMMUNOCHEMICAL METHODS FOR SERUM ALBUMIN
       MEASUREMENT   146
       12.5.1   Normal ranges   146
       12.5.2   Quality control   147

12.1   CLINICAL VALUE OF SERUM ALBUMIN MEASUREMENTS

All clinical interest is centred on low serum albumin values which may be the result of decreased synthesis, increased loss or deficient protein intake. In any pathological condition one or more of these factors may be involved.

The main areas of value are discussed below.

12.1.1   Malnutrition and malabsorption

In these states, the low serum albumin may be the result of a lack of protein digestion, e.g. in cystic fibrosis where there is deficiency of pancreatic enzymes and in malnutrition where there are insufficient amino acids to ensure an adequate supply of enzymes. The serum albumin level has been used as a standard test to confirm kwashiorkor and to monitor its response to treatment[1,2].

A low serum albumin level may be the result of a lack of absorptive mucosa, e.g. after gross surgery, resection or in severe coeliac disease. Hypoalbuminaemia has also been shown in patients with coeliac sprue[3], the reduced albumin levels being found in patients not on a gluten-free diet.

12.1.2   Protein-losing states

Low serum albumin levels may result from protein loss through the kidneys, gut or skin. In nephrosis with protein loss through the kidneys, the low serum albumin level gives rise to oedema which cannot be mobilized by diuretics. An albumin infusion given to restore arteriovenous and lymphatic circulations and kidney function makes diuretics more effective[4]. The serum albumin level is useful therefore in predicting the outcome of diuretic therapy in nephrosis.

12.1.3 Liver disease

Since the site of albumin synthesis is the liver, any impairment of liver function may affect the serum albumin level. The liver, however, has considerable reserve capacity and damage is usually severe before the albumin level is affected.

12.1.4 Malignancy

A study of hypoalbuminaemia in 360 patients[5] showed that it was most frequently associated with a diagnosis of malignant disease. In the first Medical Research Council myeloma trial the serum albumin levels at diagnosis were found to be of prognostic value[6,7]. The patients with the lowest serum albumin levels had the poorest survival rates. It is possible that low serum albumin levels could indicate a high consumption of albumin by the tumour.

12.2 STANDARDIZATION OF SERUM ALBUMIN MEASUREMENT

Techniques are now available for the rapid and precise quantitation of albumin but this improvement in technique has not overcome the inaccuracies resulting from discrepant standardization between laboratories. Some 4 years ago, a quality control scheme was started involving the supraregional protein reference centres. The albumin results of three such quality control sera are shown in Table 12.1. Faced with these results, an attempt was made to improve albumin standardization.

A wide variety of both human and bovine albumin preparations are commercially available. These preparations are widely used as standards for albumin and total protein measurement.

TABLE 12.1 Results for the serum albumin concentration of three quality control sera obtained by four or five supraregional protein reference laboratories

Centre No.	QC1	QC2	QC3
	g/l	g/l	g/l
1	39	32	19
2	44	42	19
3	42	27	13
4	42	42	42

Two major problems are involved in albumin standardization; firstly in trying to assign an accurate value for a particular standard and secondly in assessing the suitability for use in a particular technique. The simplest method of determining the albumin concentration of a preparation would be on a simple weight basis, but this depends on absolutely pure, dry products. The nitrogen content is of no real use in assigning an accurate value because of the time needed to produce meaningful results by Kjeldahl analysis.

The use of the extinction coefficient at 280 nm (absorbance is due to aromatic amino acids, mainly tyrosine, tryptophan and phenylalanine) provides another means of estimating concentrations but the different values for the extinction coefficient of human albumin present problems.

The purity of albumin preparations is a problem because estimations of the absolute equivalents of weight by ultraviolet absorption at 280 nm, nitrogen content by Kjeldahl and chromogenicity in a standard biuret reaction all depend on pure products for meaningful answers.

A variety of albumin preparations were studied in terms of purity and suitability for use in the biuret reaction[8], bromocresol green dye binding[9], RIEP[10] and AIP[11] techniques.

12.2.1   Purity of various albumin preparations

12.2.1.1   The relationship between dry weight and albumin concentration

A known weight of each dry albumin preparation was made up volumetrically in freshly prepared saline. The optical density at 280 nm was then measured. The albumin concentration of each preparation was then calculated using an $E_{280}(1 \text{ cm}, 10 \text{ g/l})$ value of $5.8^{[12]}$ for the human preparations and $6.61^{[13]}$ for the bovine ones. This value was compared with the expected value from the dry weight. For the wet preparations, the E_{280} value was compared with the value, if any, quoted for the preparations.

12.2.1.2   The presence of protein impurities in the products

The products were tested for the presence of protein impurities by crossed immunoelectrophoresis[14] against appropriate antiwhole serum. The results of the study on the relationship between dry weight and albumin concentration and the results of the crossed immunoelectrophoresis are summarized in Table 12.2.

It can be seen that trying to assign a value to a standard on a weight per volume basis may produce a very different answer to the concentration based

TABLE 12.2   The albumin preparations studied, source, type of preparation, number of impurities (if any) and a comparison of dry weight concentration with the concentration measured by ultraviolet absorption at 280 nm

Preparation	Source	Type of preparation	Impurities detected	Weight (g/l)	E_{280} conc. (g/l)
Human 1	Hyland	Freeze dried	0	36.9	29.7
2	Hyland	Freeze dried	0	23.9	15.0
3	Pentex (Miles)	Crystalline	0	9.8	9.66
4	Pentex (Miles)	Crystalline	3	4.7	3.62
5	Pentex (Miles)	Wet	0	—	61.6
6	Pentex (Miles)	Wet	0	—	58.4
7	Hoechst	Crystalline	0	60.0	55.4
8	Hoechst	Wet	0	80.0*	79.8
9	NCCLS	Wet	0	—	40.9
Bovine 10	Hoechst	Crystalline	0	56.6	52.1
11	Armour	Wet	12	60.78†	60.1
12	NCCLS	Wet	0	—	54.6

*quoted value
†calculated from the quoted nitrogen value

on the ultraviolet absorption at 280 nm. Although 5.8 is not necessarily the correct extinction coefficient for all the human preparations, even using the lowest figure quoted in the literature of 5.3[15] there would still be a discrepancy between the observed and expected values. The source of this discrepancy is probably protein or non-protein impurities. Data from manufacturers, if available, usually shows that products contain at the most 2% non-protein impurities. However on exposure to the air dry products do absorb water. It has been shown[16] that the moisture contents of commercially available albumin preparations can range from 2.7 to 9.7%.

The presence of protein impurities makes determinations of concentration by dry weight or ultraviolet absorption at 280 nm difficult unless the impurities can be quantitated and compensated for.

12.2.2   The behaviour of various albumin preparations in the estimation of albumin and total protein

Since we are concerned with immunochemical techniques only the results obtained on the human preparations will be considered.

12.2.2.1   *The biuret reaction for total protein measurement*

With a pure albumin preparation, the total protein as measured by the biuret reaction[8] can be taken as a measure of the albumin concentration. A range of dilutions made up for each preparation and the protein concentrations measured by the biuret reaction. The optical densities obtained were then plotted against the value obtained for the preparation by ultraviolet absorption at 280 nm.

12.2.2.2   *Bromocresol green dye binding (BCG)*

Although we are concerned in the main with immunochemical techniques, it is worth considering the performance of different albumin preparations in the BCG method in view of its popularity.

Using a manual BCG method[9] the albumin preparations were estimated over a range of concentrations. The optical densities of the solutions were then plotted against the E_{280} concentration for each preparation.

12.2.2.3   *Rocket immunoelectrophoresis (RIEP) and the automated immunoprecipitin (AIP) techniques*

The same batch of sheep antihuman albumin antiserum was used in both methods. A range of dilutions was made up for each preparation. After the run[11] and after processing in the case of RIEP[10] the peak heights were measured and plotted against the E_{280} concentration for each preparation.

The study on the behaviour of different albumin preparations in various methods showed that in the same method, different preparations behaved in different ways. In the biuret reaction, albumin preparations from the same manufacturer, e.g. preparations 7 and 8, and 3 and 4 agreed well with each other suggesting that some of the differences in reactivity in the biuret could be due to different source material, preparation, storage or preservative. Differences in reactivity were also apparent in the BCG dye binding method and it would appear that preparations 7 and 8 bind more dye per unit weight of albumin than preparations 5 and 6. Again preparations from the same manufacturer showed good agreement with each other.

The albumin preparations gave linear standard curves by RIEP with the exception of preparation 8 (as this preparation had the highest albumin concentration, the peak may not have been at completion). The preparations all produced different curves even when from the same manufacturer. It may be that immunochemical techniques are more sensitive to small changes in structure induced by the method of preparation of storage than chemical ones. The AIP technique also gave linear standard curves and as with RIEP all the preparations gave different curves.

12.2.3 The choice of a suitable preparation for use as a standard

Ideally the albumin preparation selected as a standard should be exactly defined in terms of its source, method of preparation, fatty acid content, and so on. The NCCLS Working Group on human serum albumin[17] decided that at the present time it was only feasible to specify the mode of preparation, purity and packaging of the standard.

From the study of various albumin preparations (by no means a comprehensive survey) a decision had to be made as to which preparation to use. Preparation 7 (Behringwerke 100% electrophoretically pure albumin ORHA 04) was chosen because of (a) its purity (which was within the NCCLS recommendations), (b) it showed the smallest discrepancy between dry weight and concentration by absorption at 280 nm and (c) it gave linear standard curves in all the methods. A final check was made on this product by determining its E_{280} (1 cm, 10 g/l). Although it must be appreciated that such measurements require considerable time to produce accurate results, a figure of 5.77 was obtained which is in good agreement with the manufacturer's data and Schönenberger's figure[12].

This method of assessing a standard is by no means ideal. What is really required is an exactly characterized human albumin preparation with a value assigned to it for international use. It has been suggested[18] that the measurement of the optical density at 280 nm does not, by itself appear to be a valid measure of the protein concentration if the preparation is to be used in immunochemical techniques. In this study, it was found that the differences

TABLE 12.3   The effect of providing the same antiserum and standard and using the same method on the measurement of albumin in five sera

Centre No.	Serum a	Serum b	Serum c	Serum d	Serum e
1	30.5	38	28	17	27
2	37	40	30	18	30
3	33	38	25	17	28
4	29	36	25	15	26
5	27	35	27	15	26

in reactivity of different preparations were no greater in the immunochemical than in the chemical techniques. Provided that the behaviour of the preparation in the method of choice is also investigated, the E_{280} method of determining albumin concentration would appear to be reasonable.

Table 12.3 shows the results obtained by the five supraregional centres when provided with standard (preparation 7) and antiserum and requested to estimate the four sera by RIEP. These results show a considerable improvement over those in Table 12.1 suggesting that some of the discrepancies between these laboratories could be due to differences in standards and possibly antiserum.

12.3   PROBLEMS WITH ALBUMIN ANALYSIS

12.3.1   Chemical methods

Although albumin is the specific protein most frequently estimated in serum, some of the routine methods of albumin analysis are far from satisfactory. The main chemical methods for albumin estimation are salt fractionation, electrophoresis and dye binding.

Salt fractionation is now rarely encountered as a means of estimating albumin. The main problem with this method (of which there are several variations) is that no matter which globulin precipitant is used there is always loss of albumin into the precipitate or incomplete globulin precipitation[19].

Electrophoresis followed by the fixation and staining of the proteins and then quantitation of the fractions by scanning or elution is a common method of albumin measurement. The sources of error in such techniques have been discussed fully elsewhere[19]. The main problems are associated with the initial estimation of the total protein and unequal dye binding of the albumin and globulin fractions. The use of correction factors to compensate for the latter is unsatisfactory[20] since they vary from serum to serum.

Albumin concentration can be estimated by the colour changes occurring in appropriate dyes when they become bound to protein. These are the dye binding methods and the ease with which they can be automated has made them the most popular methods for the estimation of albumin. Methyl orange and HABA (2,4'-hydroxyazobenzene benzoic acid) are now little used because of problems experienced with certain pathological sera and interfering substances[21,22]. Bromocresol green (BCG) is now the most widely used dye and was thought to be specific; however it has been shown the BCG reacts with non-albumin components[23,24]. Albumin levels in severely hypoalbuminaemic sera are often overestimated by BCG analysis when compared with results obtained by an immunochemical technique[19]. It is therefore in those very sera where an estimation of the albumin concentration is most important clinically that BCG analysis are the least reliable.

12.3.2 Immunochemical methods

Immunochemistry would appear to be the answer to the problem associated with the non-specificity of the chemical methods of albumin measurement. Fast specific methods are needed and the two considered are RIEP and the AIP system. Laser nephelometery would also appear to be suitable but was not included in this study. A common fault of method evaluation is that often only normal sera are used. It was considered essential to test the suitability of the RIEP and AIP methods for albumin measurement using normal and pathological sera.

12.3.2.1   Method comparison

Four groups of sera were considered, normal, cirrhotic, nephrotic and paraproteinaemic (the last three groups being chosen since it is in these conditions that albumin levels may be needed clinically and the levels may be low, the problem area for BCG). Albumin estimations in the sera of 14 patients with nephrosis, cirrhosis and paraproteinaemias using the RIEP and AIP methods

TABLE 12.4   A comparison of the RIEP and AIP techniques for albumin measurement with the radioactive albumin method using 14 pathological sera

	Correlation coefficient	Slope	Intercept
RIEP	0.98	+	*
AIP	0.98	+	*

$p < 0.001$ for both correlation coefficients
\+ not significantly different from 1.0
* not significantly different from 0

TABLE 12.5   Within batch and batch to batch variation of the RIEP and AIP methods for serum albumin measurement

	No. of measurements	Mean	Standard deviation	Coefficient of variation
RIEP				
Within batch	30	40.2	0.69	1.7
Batch to batch	50	41.1	1.15	2.7
AIP				
Within batch	30	43.0	0.73	1.7
Batch to batch	50	38.4	0.80	2.0

were compared with those using the radioactive labelled albumin method of Lubran and Moss[25]. The results of this comparison can be seen in Table 12.4. The correlation between the methods is excellent. Larger numbers of sera were then studied and other methods of albumin estimation included namely single radial immunodiffusion, an automated BCG method, electrophoresis and salt fractionation. The details of this comparison are described elsewhere[11,19,26]. Single radial immunodiffusion, BCG, electrophoresis and salt fractionation were found to be unsatisfactory, and discussion here will concentrate on the results obtained from the AIP and RIEP methods. Studies had shown that the precision of the two techniques was very similar (Table 12.5). When the two methods were compared, in all groups of sera except the paraproteinaemic group, the correlation was good (Table 12.6). Sera containing paraproteins gave significantly lower values by AIP than by RIEP ($p < 0.001$).

TABLE 12.6   A comparison of the RIEP with the AIP technique of albumin measurement in four groups of sera

	Correlation coefficient	Slope	Intercept
RIEP vs. AIP			
Normal	0.93	+	*
Cirrhotic	0.91	+	*
Nephrotic	0.85	+	*
Paraproteinaemic	0.81	+	10.1

$p < 0.001$ for all correlation coefficients
+ not significantly different from 1.0
* not significantly different from 0

12.4   THE CHOICE OF METHOD FOR ALBUMIN ANALYSIS

The main difference between the AIP and RIEP methods in terms of suit-ability for use in a routine laboratory is one of optimal batch size. RIEP as part of a busy routine laboratory could become very time-consuming over 20 to 25 samples plus standards per batch. With the AIP system the number of specimens makes little difference to the time needed to perform the assay. However the speed of the AIP system must be balanced against the high initial capital outlay for equipment, the need for monospecific antiserum of better quality and in larger quantities than required for RIEP together with the cost of servicing equipment (these comments also apply to laser nephelometry). A disadvantage of RIEP is that it does require manual skills which in a highly automated laboratory may not be easily available. Even with RIEP, although the outlay for equipment is low, for large numbers of samples a precise auto-diluter is required and this could be a costly item.

Many laboratories, even with the evidence that BCG is not specific for albumin, may be unwilling to change to immunochemical methods. This is understandable if specimen numbers are large and there is no capital for automated immunochemical equipment. Here a compromise is needed. All sera could be estimated by BCG and then sera with values say below 30 g/l estimated by RIEP. Normal albumin values are less likely to be affected by the non-specific binding of other proteins by BCG than low values. Ideally each laboratory should find out the value below which it is advisable to measure albumins immunochemically. However, this approach does present problems since one will end up with no albumin values in a certain area, say between 25 and 30 g/l. The use of two methods for serum albumin determination would necessitate two 'normal' ranges.

Another way of tackling the problem would be to measure only the albumin levels needed clinically rather than including albumin in biochemical profiles such as those produced by multichannel analysers. This move would probably meet with resistance from clinicians.

In summary, providing the number of specimens is not too large, RIEP would appear to be the method of choice for albumin measurement. It is relatively cheap both in initial outlay and recurrent expenditure on equipment and reagents. All groups of pathological sera can be measured successfully and different types of body fluid can be analysed on the same plate, e.g. serum, CSF and urine.

12.5 PROBLEMS ASSOCIATED WITH CHANGING TO IMMUNOCHEMICAL METHODS FOR SERUM ALBUMIN MEASUREMENT

12.5.1 Normal ranges

With any new method, its introduction into routine use should be preceded by the establishment of a new normal range for that method. Since the immunochemical methods of albumin determination are more specific than the dye binding ones, the normal range will tend to be lower; 197 normal sera were obtained from blood donors (ranging in age from 18 to 64 years) attending for their first donation. Blood was taken without stasis at the end of the donation (the validity of using the last blood from the donation had been tested[26]. The sera were assayed for albumin by AIP and the normal ranges obtained are shown in Table 12.7. These ranges are considerably lower than most published ranges and clinicians would have to be made fully aware of this should the laboratory contemplate changing from a dye binding method to an immunochemical method for serum albumin.

TABLE 12.7 Normal ranges for serum albumin in 197 sera measured by AIP

	−2 SD	Mean	+2 SD
Males	30	36	42
Females	27	34	42

12.5.2 Quality control

With most laboratories using BCG dye binding methods, results for albumin in quality control schemes may be precise but are not necessarily accurate. A laboratory changing to an immunochemical method would move away from the group mean albumin value. Many quality control sera are not of human origin and these are of no value for monitoring immunochemical methods.

Despite these problems, the clinical need for accurate albumin measurement coupled with the non-specificity of BCG seems to make the change to immunochemical techniques for albumin quantitation worthwhile.

Acknowledgements

I would like to thank the staff, past and present of the Protein Reference Unit, Westminster Hospital where this work was done, for their assistance and encouragement.

References

1. Truswell, A. S., Wannenberg, P., Wittman, W. and Hansen, J. D. L. (1966). Plasma amino acids in kwashiorkor. *Lancet*, **i**, 1162
2. *Lancet* (1972). Laboratory tests in protein-calorie malnutrition. *Lancet*, **i**, 1041
3. Cluysenaer, O. J. J., Corstens, F. H. M., Hafkenscheid, J. C. M., Yapp, S. H. and Von Togeren, J. H. M. (1974). *Coeliac Disease*, W. Th. J. M. Hekkens and H. E. Pena (eds.), pp. 386. (Leiden: Stenfert Kroese)
4. Chamberlain, M. J., Pringle, A. and Wrong, O. M. (1966). Oliguric renal failure in the nephrotic syndrome. *Q.J. Med.*, **35**, 215
5. Meindok, H. (1967). Diagnostic significance of hypoalbuminaemia. *J. Am. Geriatr. Soc.*, **15**, 1067
6. Peto, R. (1971). Urea, albumin and response rates. *Br. Med. J.*, **2**, 324

7. Carter, P. M., Slater, L., Lee, J., Perry, D. and Hobbs, J. R. (1975). Protein analysis in myelomatosis. *J. Clin. Pathol.*, **28** (Suppl. 6), 45
8. Gornall, A. G., Bardawill, C. J. and David, M. M. (1949). Determination of serum proteins by means of biuret reaction. *J. Biol. Chem.*, **177**, 751
9. Bartholomew, R. J. and Delaney, A. (1964). Sulphophthaleins as specific reagents for albumin; determination of albumin in serum. *Proc. Aust. Assoc. Clin. Biochem.*, **1**, 214
10. Laurell, C.-B. (1966). Quantitative estimation of proteins by electrophoresis in agarose gel containing antibodies. *Analyt. Biochem.*, **15**, 45
11. Smith, L. (1978). Albumin. In R. F. Ritchie (ed.). *Automated Immunoanalysis, Part I.* pp. 181–201 (New York: Marcel Dekker Inc.)
12. Schonenberger, V. M. (1955). Streulichtmessungen an Plasmaproteinen. *Z. Naturforsch.*, **10b**, 474
13. Peters, T. Jr. (1970). Serum albumin. *Adv. Clin. Chem.*, **13**, 37
14. Weeke, B. (1973). Crossed immunoelectrophoresis. *Scand. J. Immunol.*, **2** (Suppl. 1), 47
15. Cohn, E. J., Hughes, W. L. Jr. and Weare, J. H. (1947). Preparation and properties of serum and plasma proteins, XIII. Crystallization of serum albumin from ethanol-water mixtures. *J. Am. Chem. Soc.*, **69**, 1753
16. Doumas, B. T., Watson, W. A. and Biggs, H. G. (1971). Albumin standards and the measurement of serum albumin with bromocresol green. *Clin. Chim. Acta*, **31**, 87
17. NCCLS Working Group on Human Serum Albumin (1972). Summary of findings from the meeting held at the National Bureau of Standards, May 1972
18. Farrance, I., Dennis, P. M., Gibson, B. J. and Biegler, B. (1978). A comparative study of commercial human and bovine albumin preparations. *Ann. Clin. Biochem.*, **15**, 31
19. Slater, L., Carter, P. M. and Hobbs, J. R. (1975). Measurement of albumin in the sera of patients. *Ann. Clin. Biochem.*, **12**, 33
20. Martin, N. H. (1952). Paper strip electrophoresis. *Lancet*, **i**, 762
21. Keyser, J. W. (1968). Determination of serum albumin. *Clin. Chem.*, **14**, 360
22. Arvan, D. A. and Ritz, A. (1969). Measurement of albumin by the H.A.B.A. dye technique. A study of the effect of free and conjugated bilirubin, of bile acids and of certain drugs. *Clin. Chim. Acta*, **26**, 505
23. Webster, D., Bignell, A. H. C. and Attwood, E. C. (1974). An assessment of the suitability of bromocresol green for the determination of serum albumin. *Clin. Chim. Acta*, **53**, 101
24. Webster, D. (1974). A study of the interaction of bromocresol green with isolated serum globulin fractions. *Clin. Chim. Acta*, **53**, 109
25. Lubran, M. and Moss, D. W. (1957). The determination of serum albumin concentration using ^{131}I-labelled albumin. *Clin. Chim. Acta*, **2**, 246
26. Slater, L. (1975). The determination of specific protein values in normal and abnormal sera with special reference to immunochemical assays. PhD. thesis. University of London

13

The complement system

J. T. Whicher

13.1	INTRODUCTION	150
13.2	PHYSIOLOGY OF THE COMPLEMENT SYSTEM	151
	13.2.1 The classical pathway	153
	13.2.2 The alternative pathway	154
13.3	LABORATORY MEASUREMENT OF COMPLEMENT	156
	13.3.1 Functional assays	156
	13.3.2 Immunochemical assays for complement components	157
	13.3.3 Immunochemical detection of complement activation products	157
13.4	COMPLEMENT AND DISEASE	157
13.5	COMPLEMENT MEASUREMENTS IN DISEASE	158
	13.5.1 Inherited deficiencies of complement components	158
	13.5.2 Inherited deficiencies of complement inhibitors	159
	13.5.3 Complement as an indicator system in immune complex disease	160
	13.5.4 Complement as an indicator of alternative pathway activity	161
13.6	BIOLOGICAL PROBLEMS IN THE USE OF COMPLEMENT MEASUREMENTS	162
13.7	WHAT TESTS SHOULD BE USED AND WHEN?	162

13.1 INTRODUCTION

The humoral immune defence mechanism eliminates antigens by a number of effector pathways. All these pathways are dependent upon either the generation of active sites in the Fc region of antibody molecules or immunoglobulin aggregation generated by antigen binding. Such sites interact either directly or *via* the complement system with specialized cells which are responsible for the process of inflammation and antigen removal.

(a) Activated Fc of immunoglobulin will bind to receptors on:

platelets—causing release of nucleotides and amines

neutrophils—resulting in phagocytosis and release of proteolytic enzymes

eosinophils—which may become cytotoxic

basophils and mast cells—resulting in degranulation

mononuclear phagocytes—causing phagocytosis or contact lysis

K (killer) cells—causing antibody-dependent cell-mediated cytolysis.

(b) Activated Fc of immunoglobulin will activate complement, resulting in:

immune adherence—neutrophils bind to cell membranes bearing activated complement; exocytosis of granules and phagocytosis then occurs

chemotaxis—migration of leukocytes towards complement components released into the fluid phase

anaphylatoxin activity—activated complement released into the fluid phase causes degranulation of mast cells

lysis of cells—cell-membrane bound complement results in membrane permeability.

Antibody and complement together result in a sophisticated and integrated antigen elimination system. Complement is important as it can be seen that the free fluid phase activities of the humoral immune system are complement mediated, as is lysis.

The defence mechanism depends upon phagocytosis and in some cases lysis, facilitated by important alterations in the surrounding tissues. The sequence of events may be summarized as follows (Figure 13.1):

(a) Tissue is invaded by antigen. If specific antibody is present complement effector molecules are produced. These cause histamine release from mast cells resulting in smooth muscle contraction and vascular permeability. Oedema and stasis result with passage of further antibody and complement into the infected extravascular space.

(b) The spread of infection is limited by thrombosis of surrounding blood vessels due to platelet aggregation and intravascular coagulation.

(c) Complement-derived chemotaxins result in migration of phagocytes into the area.

(d) Phagocytes and killer cells adhere to the antigen by receptors for Fc and complement with proteolytic destruction and phagocytosis of the foreign material.

(e) Cellular antigens may be lysed by the complement system.

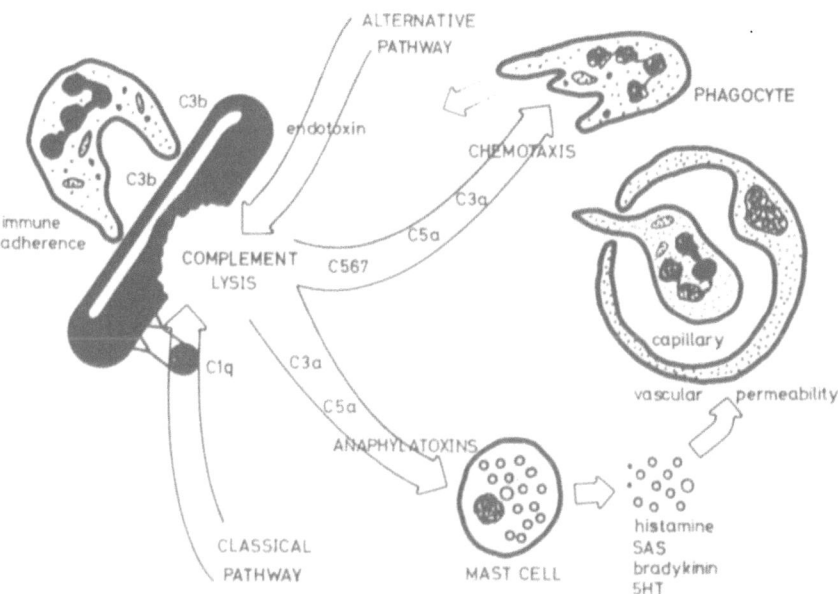

Figure 13.1 The role of complement in the defence against microorganisms. Only the most important functions are shown

13.2 PHYSIOLOGY OF THE COMPLEMENT SYSTEM

Complement is clearly an important part of the *adaptive* immune response. The pathway of this molecular interaction with Fc of antibody is called the *classical pathway*. Complement may however interact directly with certain antigens, notably bacterial lipopolysaccharide, to activate all its biological effector mechanisms via the *alternative pathway*. This mechanism of immediate or non-adaptive immune defence is extremely important.

The complement system comprises a group of proteins which, following activation, interact with each other in a sequential fashion to produce biological effector molecules. The individual protein components share a number of important properties:

(a) The sequential activation often results in proteolytic cleavage of components by the ones preceding them in the sequence. The products are referred to as activation of conversion products.

(b) Such cleavage may result in the appearance of binding sites for other complement proteins, thus allowing assembly of component complexes.

(c) Activated components may possess binding sites for cell membranes, thus causing transfer from the fluid phase to sites on the cell membrane. The activated binding sites rapidly decay, constituting an important control mechanism.

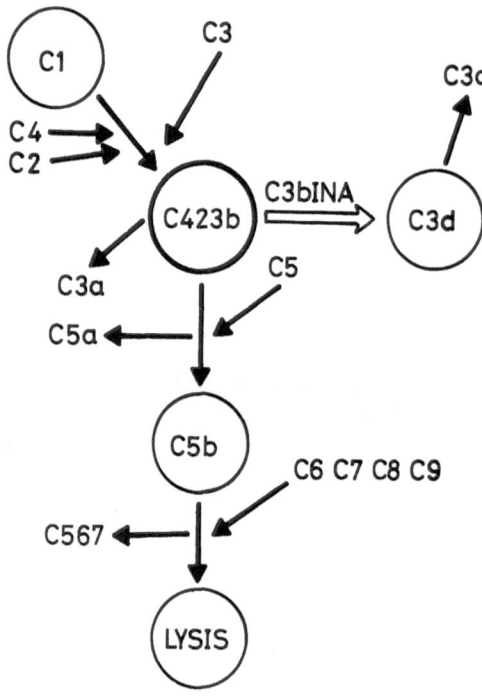

Figure 13.2 The classical pathway of complement activation. Antigen–antibody complexes activate C1 which initiates a proteolytic cascade, generating C5b onto which C6–C9 assemble to form the lytic complex. Cell-bound C3b, for which many cells have receptors, is destroyed by C3b inactivator (C3bINA) producing C3d which is cell bound and has residual immune adherence function and C3c an inactive fluid phase component. Fluid phase effector molecules are produced (C3a, C5a and C567). Only the biologically important fragments are shown

In essence, the system is a proteolytic cascade, resulting in assembly of protein molecules on cell membranes with the release of low molecular weight cleavage fragments, possessing biological effector activity. The molecular dynamics of the two pathways of complement activation will be briefly summarized. For more detailed descriptions see references 1, 3–5.

13.2.1 The classical pathway (Figure 13.2)

Activation of the classical pathway is initiated by the binding of the C1 macro-molecule (comprising C1q, C1r and C1s, held together by calcium ions) to two critically spaced activated Fc regions. The chances of two randomly placed IgG molecules being at this critical distance is low (0.5×10^6 molecules on a red cell would be required to activate one C1q molecule). IgG is thus an inefficient complement activator. The Fc regions of pentameric IgM are how-ever already critically spaced; thus one IgM molecule can activate one C1q molecule.

Activation of C1s exposes an active site which is able to cleave C4 and C2 into two fragments and bind to the major portions (Figure 13.3). The C42 complex is released from C1 and binds to the cell membrane, thereby releasing C1s for further C4 and C2 cleavage resulting in *amplification*. C42 cleaves C3 into two fragments, C3a with anaphylatoxic and chemotactic activity and C3b for which leukocytes have immune adherence receptors. C3b is cell bound

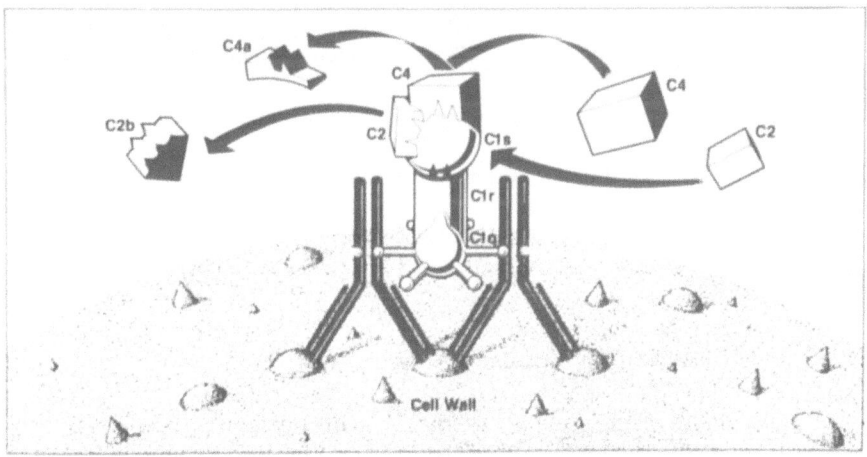

Figure 13.3 The activation of C1 by the Fc of two critically-spaced IgG molecules with the subsequent cleavage of C4 and C2

and is responsible for proteolytic cleavage of C5, C5a has similar effector functions to C3a, and C5b remains cell bound. C6 binds to C5b and components C6 to C9 assemble without cleavage, generating the lytic complex, which results in hole-like ultra-structural lesions in the cell membrane. A free fluid phase C567 complex is produced which is a chemotaxin.

C3 is of central importance as it is at this point that the major control enzyme (C3b inactivator, C3b INA) exerts its effect (there are a number of other inactivators of which C1 inactivator, C1 INH, is clinically important). C3 also generates several of the complement effector molecules (Table 13.1). It is at the level of C3 that the alternative pathway enters the system and that an important positive feedback loop operates (in which C423b may participate).

TABLE 13.1 Complement effector molecules

Function	Component	Cells affected
Immune adherence	C3b C3d C4b	Primate erythrocytes, non-primate platelets, macrophages, polymorpho-nuclear leukocytes, B-lymphocytes
Chemotaxins	C3a C5a C567	Polymorphonuclear leukocytes, macrophages and eosinophils
Anaphylatoxicity	C3a C5a	Mast cells and basophils
Exocytosis of neutrophil granules	C3b C5a	Polymorphonuclear leukocytes
Vascular permeability (kinin-like action)	C2 fragment	Capillary endothelial cells
Leukocyte mobilization from the bone marrow	C3 fragment	Polymorphonuclear leukocytes
Membrane lesions	C5–C9 complex	Any cells

13.2.2   The alternative pathway (Figure 13.4)

The molecular dynamics of the alternative pathway are both complex and open to controversy, and a simplified version will be presented here. The pathway activates the terminal components of the classical pathway from C3 to C9. It may be activated by a wide range of substances, the most important

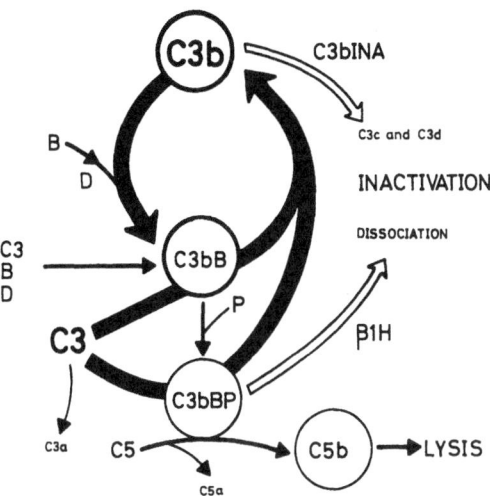

Figure 13.4 The alternative pathway of complement activation. The pathway is activated by the protection of C3b from C3bINA and of C3bBP from β1H, thus allowing the positive feedback loop to accelerate. The cycle is maintained by the low-level spontaneous production of C3bB from C3 and B in the presence of Mg^{2+} and D[6]

of which are probably bacterial lipopolysaccharides. It is thus responsible for the immediate defence against invading organisms, not requiring the relatively slow process of antibody formation and, as such, appears to be an extremely important defence mechanism.

The alternative pathway comprises a continuously cycling positive feedback loop. C3b combines with Factor B in the presence of magnesium and Factor D to form a complex C3bB, which may be stabilized by the addition of properdin (P). Both C3bB and C3bBP are able to activate native C3 to form C3b, which in turn combines with Factor B in the presence of magnesium. C3bBP is also a C5 convertase. The cycle is controlled by the removal of C3b by C3bINA, either directly or after dissociation of the C3bB and C3bBP complexes by the protein β1H. Clearly anything that generates C3b activates the cycle. Two theories prevail for the mechanism of activation:

(a) It is suggested that C3bB is being generated all the time by the low grade assembly of C3 and B in the presence of D. The 'activating' substance has the capacity to protect the C3b from C3INA and C3bBP from β1H, thus allowing the feedback loop to 'accelerate'[6].

(b) Muller-Eberhard's group[7] have suggested that a serum factor, 'initiating factor (IF), is activated and combines with Factor B and C3 to form a complex IFBC3 which is able to convert C3 to C3b, thus providing input for the feedback loop. However, Fearon[6] suggests that IF (or C3 nephritic factor) acts by protecting C3bB from the action of β1H. C423b generated from the classical pathway C3 convertase will also provide input for the loop, but it does not appear as active as when true alternative pathway activation is occurring. This tends to support the first hypothesis that alternative pathway activation works by protecting C3b.

13.3   LABORATORY MEASUREMENT OF COMPLEMENT

The laboratory measurement of complement is aimed at:

(a) The detection of genetic defects within the complement system. This may be a homozygous deficiency with no detectable components, a heterozygous deficiency with low levels or a defective component present in normal concentration.

(b) The detection of complement activation as an indication that complement is involved in a pathological process.

The types of measurement available are:

(a) Functional assays dependent upon the generation of effector molecules, e.g. haemolytic assays or opsonization assays.

(b) Immunochemical assays measuring individual component concentrations.

(c) Immunochemical detection and possibly measurement of products of complement activation, e.g. C3a or C4d.

13.3.1   Functional assays

These are essential when investigating genetic complement defects. Simple haemolytic assays are available for the integrity of the whole classical or alternative pathways, which form useful screening procedures. Specific haemolytic assays for all the classical pathway components are also available. Tests for other biological effector molecules have been described but are more difficult to perform. Functional assays can have a high degree of specificity but poor sensitivity, and are expensive in time and reagents.

13.3.2   Immunochemical assays for complement components

Antibodies to most complement proteins have now been produced and quantitative immunochemical techniques such as radial immunodiffusion, Laurell rocket immunoelectrophoresis, continuous flow and discreet nephelometry can be used to measure them. There are two important limitations to the use of these measurements as an indicator system for complement activation:

(a) During the process of complement activation, several complement components are consumed, lowering their plasma levels. However, they are acute phase proteins (see below) and synthesis increases, tending to normalize levels.

(b) During complement activation low molecular weight fragments are produced, which result in overestimation of levels of some components (C3 and C4) by radial immunodiffusion and Laurell rocket immunoelectrophoresis. This will give rise to an overestimation in just those situations in which low levels are being sought. Activation of complement *in vitro* easily occurs and causes similar problems. This can largely be avoided by simple precautions, including the use of EDTA in samples[8].

13.3.3   Immunochemical detection of complement activation products

The activation products of C3, C4 and Factor B are separable from the native molecule on the basis of their different sizes and charges, and may thus be detected by immunoelectrophoresis or crossed immunoelectrophoresis[9]. Antisera to some of these activation products are becoming available[10].

The detection of activation products is the most sensitive technique available for assessing complement involvement in disease, but it is crucial that activation *in vitro* does not occur.

13.4   COMPLEMENT AND DISEASE

Complement is the main effector mechanism of the humoral immune response and as such is responsible for much of the damage caused when antibodies are directed against host tissues, for example in transfusion reactions or autoimmune haemolytic anaemias. Complement may also damage host cells when antibody–antigen complexes become passively deposited on them from the blood or extravascular fluid. The activation of complement is a physiological process but damages host cells as a result of pathological deposition of immune complexes on them. Such diseases usually reflect the deposition of complexes from the blood stream, in which case it is the vascular endothelial cells which take the brunt of the damage. Similar damage may occur when complexes are present in extravascular fluid, such as synovial fluid or CSF.

It is becoming clear that an increased susceptibility to infections may result from genetic deficiencies of complement components.

A number of inactivating enzymes are known to act as control mechanisms in the complement pathway. Their inherited deficiency may also give rise to disease as a result of spontaneous activation of the complement system.

13.5   COMPLEMENT MEASUREMENTS IN DISEASE

Complement measurements may be used for a number of rather different purposes:

(a) To detect inherited deficiencies giving rise to infection.

(b) To detect inherited deficiencies of inhibitors, giving rise to damage to tissues as a result of spontaneous activation.

(c) As an indicator system to detect and monitor diseases due to the deposition of immune complexes within the vascular system. (Deposition of complexes locally in tissue does not usually give rise to measurable complement alternations in the plasma, though it may do so in fluids such as CSF or synovial fluid).

(d) As an indicator system to detect pathological processes resulting in alternative pathway activation of complement.

13.5.1   Inherited deficiencies of complement components

Genetic deficiencies of most of the complement components have now been described[11,12]. Several interesting aspects concerning the role of the complement system in the overall immune defence mechanism have arisen from these studies and allow the division of these diseases into a number of groups:

(a) Deficiencies of the early part of the classical pathway. C1, C4 and C2 have been associated with immune complex disease, predominantly syndromes like systemic lupus erythematosus (SLE). There may be a genuine aetiological relationship or this may be due to an ascertainment artefact.

(b) Deficiencies of the alternative pathway have not been clearly described, but there are a number of patients with severe bacterial infection in whom activation *in vitro* of the alternative pathway by bacterial lipopolysaccharide is defective.

(c) Deficiencies of C3 and C3INA. In the absence of C3bINA the C3b feedback loop in uninhibited and C3 is consumed. In both these conditions, severe infections result, probably due to an absence of most of the biological effector molecules.

(d) Deficiencies of the C5 to C9 sequence have shown a striking association with neisserial infections and it is thus possible that lysis is important in elimination of these organisms.

The inferences that may be drawn from these findings are that the early classical pathway is relatively unimportant in defence against infection except perhaps for viruses, which may be implicated in such immune complex diseases as SLE. The alternative pathway and C3 are very important. The lytic sequence is probably only important against some types of organism.

Many of the defects described are *functional* with normal immunochemically measured component concentrations. It is thus crucial in the investigation of genetic complement deficiencies that functional assays are used. It is also clear that some effector molecules may be defective whilst others are normal. For example, cases have been seen where lysis is normal but opsonization is not. The serious investigation of complement deficiencies is a very complex problem, requiring a range of functional bioassays.

13.5.2   Inherited deficiencies of complement inhibitors

C1 esterase inhibitor (C1INA) deficiency or hereditary angioneurotic oedema is the commonest inherited deficiency within the complement system. The patients suffer from recurrent attacks of peripheral, bronchial and gastrointestinal oedema. The spontaneous activation of C1 occurs with consumption of C4 and C2; C3 and later components are unaffected. It is probable that C1 activation is caused by proteolytic digestion of C1 by plasmin, for which C1INA is an important inhibitor. The oedema is caused by a vascular permeability-inducing peptide released from C2; 80% of patients have low levels (10–20% if normal) of C1INA. In these people the inheritance is dominant which, together with the detectable levels of C1INA, suggests that these are in fact heterozygotes; 20% of patients have normal immunochemically-measured levels of C1INA, but with a poorly functional protein. A functional assay is thus essential in investigating this disease.

C3INA deficiency has already been mentioned because it gives rise to effective C3 deficiency as a result of consumption by the uninhibited cycling of the feedback loop. Patients also suffer from skin itching due to histamine release generated by C3a.

13.5.3 Complement as an indicator system in immune complex disease

A classification of immune complex diseases is given in Table 13.2[13]. Immune complexes in plasma may be measured directly by a wide variety of methods, varying enormously in their specificity and sensitivity[14]. Evidence of complement activation may be used to infer the *active deposition* of immune complexes. Clearly this gives very different information from direct measurement, but is useful because complement activation *in vivo* implies active disease, provides a pointer to pathogenesis and may be quantitatively related to tissue damage.

Complement measurement may thus be used to answer the question of whether a particular disease or symptom complex is likely to be due to immune

TABLE 13.2   A classification of some immune complex diseases

Disease	Antigen
Exogenous antigens	
polyarteritis nodosa	?viral
hepatitis B	viral
post-streptococcal glomerulonephritis	bacterial
subacute bacterial endocarditis	bacterial
'shunt' nephritis	bacterial
malarial nephritis	protozoal
serum sickness	foreign proteins
drug allergy	drug-protein complex
Endogenous antigens	
rheumatoid arthritis	immunoglobulin
mixed cryoglobulinaemia	immunoglobulin
systemic lupus erythematosus	nuclear material
Unknown antigens	
much chronic glomerulonephritis and vasculitis	

TABLE 13.3   Diseases in which complement assays are of value in diagnosis or treatment in Europe*

	Disease	Investigations
Inborn errors of complement metabolism	C1 esterase inhibitor deficiency	Functional and immunochemical assay of C1 inhibitor
	Monocomponent deficiencies	Total haemolytic complement functional and immunochemical assays of components
Systemic immune complex disease	Systemic lupus erythematosus	Decreased C4 level with C3 conversion products present are the most reliable tests
	Rheumatoid vasculitis	Decreased C3 with C3 conversion
	Polymyalgia rheumatica	C3 conversion products
	Mixed cryoglobulinaemia	C3 conversion products
	Subacute bacterial endocarditis	Decreased total C3 and C4 with conversion products
	'Shunt' nephritis	Decreased total C3 and C4 with conversion products
Glomerulonephritis	Post-streptococcal	C3 decreased with conversion products. Returns to normal in two months
	Mesangio capillary	Persistent low C3 with conversion products and normal C4. Factor B conversion products may be found
Shock syndromes	Gram-negative bacteraemia	Decreased total C3. C3 conversion products present. Normal C4 level. Decreased Factor B with conversion products

*Complement assays may be very useful in a number of tropical diseases with immune complex deposition or alternative pathway activation

complex deposition. More importantly, in a few diseases changes are clear-cut enough to base diagnosis and monitoring of treatment on them (Table 13.3).

13.5.4   Complement as an indicator of alternative pathway activity

The alternative pathway (Figure 13.4) often becomes involved in classical pathway activation due to activation of the C3b feedback loop. It is thus important that tests of alternative pathway activation are interpreted in this light.

The clinical syndrome of Gram-negative bacteraemia or septicaemia associated with shock is probably due to activation of the alternative complement pathway by bacterial endotoxin or lipopolysaccharide with subsequent involvement of platelets and disseminated intramuscular coagulation. Diagnostically, complement measurement, particularly of C3 conversion products, may be very useful in distinguishing this from other causes of post-surgical shock.

13.6   BIOLOGICAL PROBLEMS IN THE USE OF COMPLEMENT MEASUREMENTS

The evaluation of complement measurements is complicated by a number of factors *in vivo*:

(a) Many complement components behave as acute phase reactants and plasma levels rise in most inflammatory conditions. If decreased complement levels are used as a means of detecting complement involvement in disease they may well be masked by this acute phase increase.

(b) Proteolytic enzymes from necrotic tissue may give rise to complement breakdown products similar to those of immune activation.

(c) Immune complexes may be produced in showers of short duration, the clinical features of vascular damage appearing some time after the event.

13.7   WHAT TESTS SHOULD BE USED AND WHEN?

Patients with suspected inherited deficiencies in the complement system require the widest range of possible tests, including functional assays not only for components but for effector molecules.

The question often arises as to whether a symptom complex could be due to immune complex deposition. Under these circumstances, the most sensitive test is desirable. If possible, a direct test for immune complexes should be used in conjunction with a sensitive test for complement activation products, such as crossed immunoelectrophoresis for C3c. Measurement of total C3 or C4 may or may not be useful.

The detection and monitoring of the immune complex diseases in which complement measurement is of known value are shown in Table 13.3.

It may be of interest to establish whether activation of complement is occurring by the classical or by the alternative pathway. The most practical way of achieving this is to look for the presence of C3 and Factor B activation products in the absence of C4 activation. These tests may be simply performed by crossed immunoelectrophoresis.

References

1. Muller-Eberhard, H. J. (1975). Complement. *Ann. Rev. Biochem.*, **44**, 899
2. Lachmann, P. J. (1975). *The Immune System*. In Hobart, M. J. and McConnell, I. (eds.) p. 56. (Oxford: Blackwell)
3. Mayer, M. M. (1972). Mechanism of cytolysis by complement. *Proc. Nat. Acad. Sci. USA*, **69**, 2954
4. Muller-Eberhard, H. J. (1974). Patterns of complement activation. In Brent, L. and Holborrow, J. (eds.). *Progress in Immunology*, **1**, 173. (Amsterdam: North Holland Publishing Company)
5. Fearon, D. T. and Austen, F. K. (1976). The human complement system: Biochemistry, biology and pathobiology. *Essays Med. Biochem.*, **2**, 1
6. Fearon, D. T. and Austen, F. K. (1977). Activation of the alternative complement pathway with rabbit erythrocytes by circumvention of the regulatory action of endogenous control proteins. *J. Exp. Med.*, **146**, 22
7. Medicus, R. G., Schrieber, R. D., Gotze, O. and Muller-Eberhard, H. J. (1976). A molecular concept of the properdin pathway. *Proc. Nat. Acad. Sci. U.S.A.*, **73**, 612
8. Alper, C. A. and Rosen, F. S. (1975). Clinical applications of complement assays. *Adv. Int. Med.*, **20**, 61
9. Versey, J. M. B. (1973). Automated two-dimensional immunoelectrophoresis and its application to the analysis of C3 and C4 in rheumatoid arthritis and systemic lupus erythematosus (SLE). *Ann. Clin. Biochem.*, **10**, 100
10. Perrin, L. H., Lambert, P. H. and Miescher, P. A. (1975). Complement breakdown products in plasma from patients with systemic lupus erythematosus and patients with membranoproliferative or other glomerulonephritis. *J. Clin. Invest.*, **56**, 165
11. Lachmann, P. J. (1976). Clinical effects of complement deficiency. In Peters, D. K. (ed.). *Advanced Medicine*, **12**, 43. (London: Pitman Medical)
12. Soothill, J. F. and Harvey, B. A. M. (1977). A defect of the alternative pathway of complement. *Clin. Exp. Immunol.*, **27**, 30
13. World Health Organisation (1977). The role of immune complexes in disease. *Technical Report Series*, **606**, 1
14. Zubler, R. H. and Lambert, P. H. (1977). Immune complexes in clinical investigations. In Thompson, R. A. (ed.). *Recent Advances in Clinical Immunology*, **1**, 129. (Edinburgh: Churchill Livingstone)

14

Alphafetoprotein in obstetrics

D. J. H. Brock

14.1 INTRODUCTION   165

14.2 AMNIOTIC FLUID ALPHAFETOPROTEIN   166
    14.2.1 *Method of measurement*   166
    14.2.2 *Clinical use*   167
    14.2.3 *AFP and genetic counselling*   170

14.3 MATERNAL SERUM ALPHAFETOPROTEIN   171
    14.3.1 *Method of measurement*   171
    14.3.2 *Screening for neural tube defects*   171
    14.3.3 *Other abnormalities associated with elevated maternal
        serum AFP*   173
    14.3.4 *Multiple pregnancy*   174
    14.3.5 *Future prospects*   174

14.1 INTRODUCTION

The existence of a specific and distinct α_1-globulin in human fetal serum was first noted in 1956[1], and named alphafetoprotein (AFP). It is the main protein in the circulation of the early fetus, being synthesized at a rate of up to

30 mg per day in the second trimester. Concentrations of AFP in fetal blood reach a peak of 3–4 mg/ml at the 13th week of gestation, and thereafter decline. In amniotic fluid, levels of AFP closely parallel those in fetal serum but at about 1/100th of the concentration[2].

The importance of AFP in obstetrics arises primarily from its feto-specificity. Most of the protein of early amniotic fluid is maternal in origin and only AFP offers unambiguous information on the fetus. Furthermore AFP is able to enter the maternal circulation both by crossing the membranes and trans-placentally. In practice this means that fetal conditions may be monitored by simple chemical tests made on the mother's blood.

14.2 AMNIOTIC FLUID ALPHAFETOPROTEIN

14.2.1 Method of measurement

Measurements of AFP in amniotic fluid are usually made on amniocentesis samples taken between the 15th and 20th weeks of pregnancy. At this stage of gestation levels of AFP in normal samples range between 5 and 40 μg/ml. The most commonly used assay techniques for amniotic fluid AFP are the rocket electrophoresis method of Laurell and single radial immunodiffusion. Both methods are satisfactory but rocket electrophoresis is probably the more precise (Figure 14.1). High quality antisera against AFP are available com-mercially, as is an international reference standard based on human cord

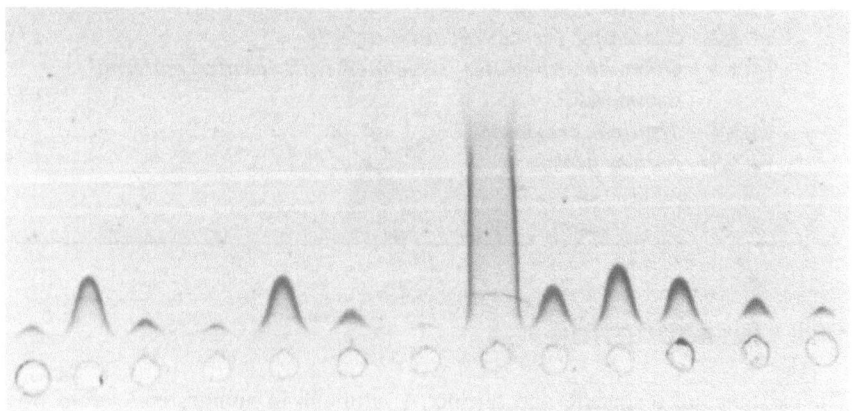

Figure 14.1   Rocket electrophoresis of amniotic fluid AFP. The open-topped rocket indicates a neural tube defect

serum. In-house standards of cord serum, calibrated against the international standard, should be maintained in the frozen state below −30 °C and discarded after use.

Amniotic fluid AFP concentrations decrease with advancing gestation, from a peak at about 13 weeks. Normal values are best expressed in terms of standard deviations above the mean for individual weeks of pregnancy (Table 14.1). Though a number of normal ranges have been published, inter-laboratory variation is considerable. Individual laboratories should therefore establish their own means and standard deviations. In doing this it is necessary to avoid the use of frozen samples, unless the degree of blood contamination in the sample has been carefully recorded. A small degree of fetal blood contamination in amniotic fluid can lead to spuriously high values.

TABLE 14.1 Normal range for amniotic fluid AFP

Gestation (weeks)	Number	Mean ± standard deviation (µg/ml)
14	30	16.7 ± 4.8
15	51	13.0 ± 5.0
16	114	11.6 ± 4.3
17	76	9.3 ± 3.8
18	41	7.9 ± 3.4
19	34	5.8 ± 2.4
20	17	4.7 ± 1.9

14.2.2 Clinical use

The main clinical use of amniotic fluid AFP measurements is in the early prenatal diagnosis of open neural tube defects. This was first introduced in 1972[3,4] and is now extensively used by laboratories offering prenatal diagnostic services. In general amniotic fluid AFP concentrations are grossly elevated with both anencephaly and open spina bifida (Figure 14.2), though some small spina bifida lesions may give more marginally increased concentrations[5]. Closed neural tube defects, represented in the main by meningocele spina bifidas and encephaloceles, are not usually associated with increases in AFP values. The closed lesions may represent between 5 and 10% of all neural tube defects.

It is now known that amniotic fluid AFP is not a specific measure in the diagnosis of neural tube defects. A number of other fetal abnormalities have been reported to be associated with increased AFP concentrations[6]. The most common of these are intrauterine death (missed abortion), exomphalos congenital nephrosis and various types of fetal teratoma. Other conditions where AFP is occasionally increased or where information from the critical second trimester of pregnancy is not as yet available, are shown in Table 14.2. It should be noted that in general all these conditions are serious and should

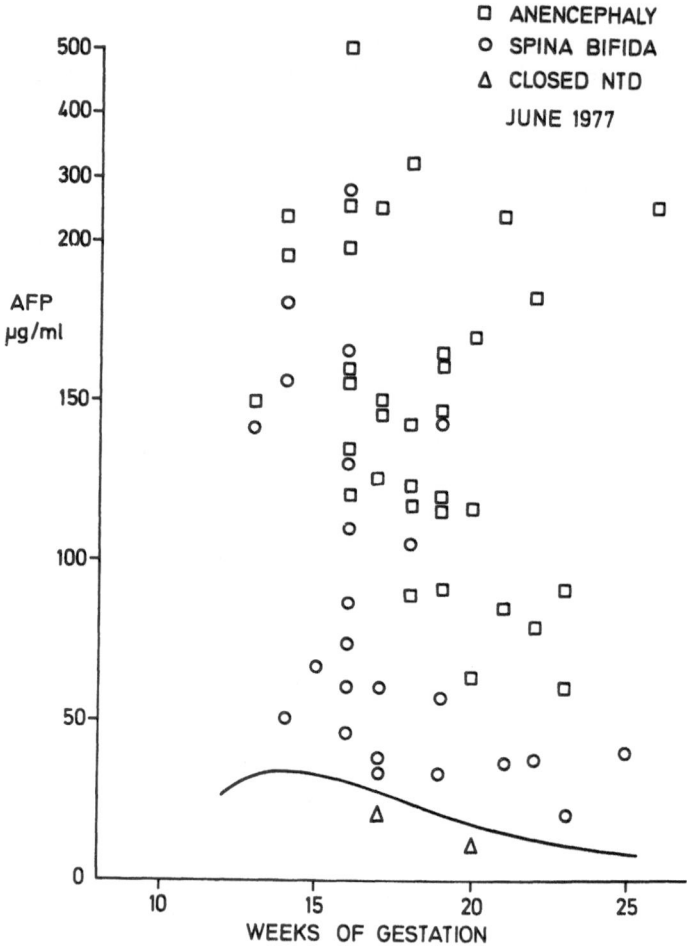

Figure 14.2 Amniotic fluid AFP concentrations for open neural tube defects. Experience from the author's laboratory to June 1977

TABLE 14.2 Conditions associated with elevated concentrations of amniotic fluid AFP

Probable	Possible
Anencephaly	Gastrointestinal atresias
Open spina bifida	Turner's syndrome
Congenital nephrosis	Meckel syndrome
Intrauterine death (missed abortion)	Polycystic kidneys
Fetal teratomas	Fallot's tetralogy
Exomphalos	Annular pancreas
	Congenital skin lesions

not compromise the use of amniotic fluid AFP in diagnosing the more common open neural tube defects.

Two technical hazards confront users of AFP in prenatal diagnosis. The first results from a misdirected amniocentesis which has produced urine from the maternal bladder rather than amniotic fluid from the amniotic sac[7]. A number of procedures have been suggested for distinguishing urine and amniotic fluid, but a complete absence of AFP in a sample should alert the laboratory technician to the possibility of a misdirected amniocentesis. The second problem is a more serious one and results from the fact that AFP concentrations in fetal serum are between 100 and 200 times the values found in amniotic fluid[2]. A comparatively small admixture of fetal blood with the amniotic fluid can increase the AFP value to a point where it mimics the values found in open neural tube defects. In many laboratories current practice is to set aside an aliquot of whole amniotic fluid from any sample where there is visible blood contamination[8]. If the AFP value is elevated the cell button can then be examined for the presence of fetal red blood cells by Kleihauer test, by electrophoresis of haemoglobin or by the use of commercial antisera directed against haemoglobin F. Contaminated samples with moderately raised AFP values, which contain a major proportion of fetal blood, should be rejected and a fresh amniocentesis called for. It must be noted that many anencephalic fetuses bleed spontaneously into the fluid. However, the AFP values associated with anencephaly are usually so high (often 20 to 100 standard deviations above the mean) that these samples are unlikely to be confused with normal samples which have been contaminated with fetal blood as a result of amniocentesis[9].

As in any other diagnostic test both false positive and false negative determinations of AFP have been reported. The proportion of these depends on the cut-off point chosen by the laboratory involved. Usually this is set

TABLE 14.3 Amniotic fluid AFP concentrations in open neural tube defects expressed in terms of standard deviations above the mean for the gestational week

Standard deviations	Open spina bifida	Anencephaly
<3	1	0
3–4	0	0
4–5	1	0
5–6	1	0
6–7	1	0
7–8	2	0
8–9	3	0
9–10	1	0
>10	32	45
Total	43	45

TABLE 14.4 Empirical risk of neural tube defect (NTD) in various family situations

Family history	Risk (%)*
One child with NTD	5
Two children with NTD	10
Parent with NTD	4.5
One child with multiple vertebral anomalies	5
One child with spinal dysraphism	4

*These risks apply only to the UK, or populations where the birth incidence of NTD is of the order of 5 per 1000

somewhere between 3 and 5 standard deviations above the mean for the gestational week in question. As shown in Table 14.3 my own choice is 4 standard deviations. However, in the absence of ancillary tests it is unlikely that there will be a single cut-off point which will absolutely distinguish the normal from the abnormal pregnancy.

14.2.3 AFP and genetic counselling

The primary causation of neural tube defects is unknown. Empirical studies show that the recurrence risk for a mother who has given birth to a child with either anencephaly or spina bifida depends on the local incidence of the defect. In the United Kingdom recurrence risks after a single affected child are of the order of 5%, while in most other parts of the world the recurrence risks are somewhat lower. Other categories of family history in which recurrence risks are known are shown in Table 14.4. Since these are all quite high it is important that the families at risk be acquainted with the facts of amniocentesis and antenatal diagnosis. It should also be noted that the Meckel syndrome, which is inherited as an autosomal recessive and where recurrence risks after an affected child are 25%, can often be diagnosed by measurement of amniotic fluid AFP[10].

14.3 MATERNAL SERUM ALPHAFETOPROTEIN

14.3.1 Method of measurement

AFP may be detected in maternal serum (or plasma) from as early as the middle of the first trimester. Concentrations rise quite sharply to a plateau at about 32 or 33 weeks of pregnancy. However, at all stages AFP values are much lower than those found in amniotic fluid and cannot be measured by techniques appropriate for amniotic fluid. Instead more sensitive procedures such as immunoautoradiography, radioimmunoelectrophoresis, enzyme-linked immunoabsorbent assay (ELISA) and radioimmunoassay (RIA) must be used. Of these radioimmunoassay is usually thought to be the most appropriate both for the ng/ml levels of AFP and for the large numbers of samples often encountered. A wide variety of RIA techniques are now available, including double-antibody, polyethylene glycol and solid phase procedures. All have their proponents and none would appear to have significant advantages over any other.

14.3.2 Screening for neural tube defects

The possibility of maternal serum AFP measurements being used in the early prediction of neural tube defects was suggested in 1972[3]. However, it was clear that it was not a diagnostic procedure, but had to be seen as a broad screening technique, to be followed where necessary by ultrasonic scan, diagnostic amniocentesis and the measurement of amniotic fluid AFP. The range of values found in normal pregnancies was extremely wide and over-lapped to a considerable degree with those found in cases of neural tube defect. Furthermore not all cases of either anencephaly or open spina bifida could be predicted from serum AFP determinations[11,12,13].

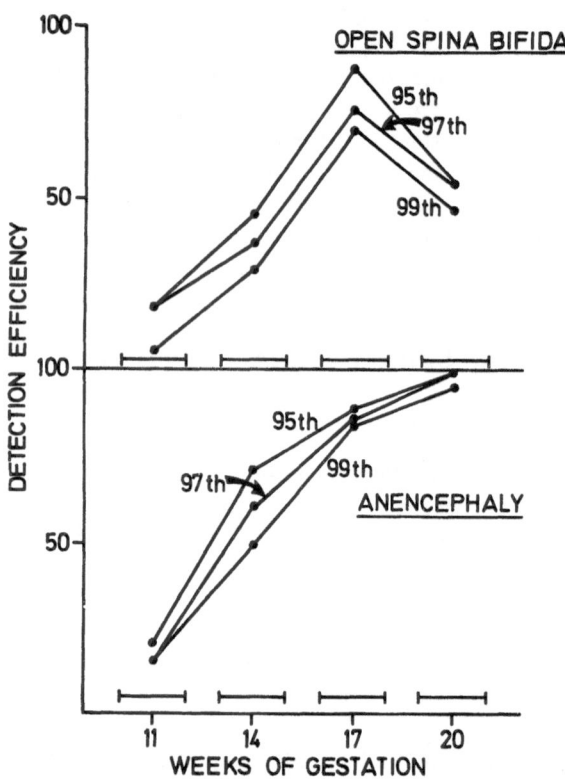

Figure 14.3 Detection efficiency for open spina bifida and anencephaly using different percentiles as cut-off points. Data from the UK Collaborative Study

The most definitive account of the potential of serum AFP screening comes from the report of the UK Collaborative Study on alphafetoprotein in relation to neural tube defects[14]. It is based on data from 19 participating laboratories and comprises serum AFP determinations from 18 684 singleton pregnancies, 163 twin pregnancies and 288 pregnancies where the fetus had an open neural tube defect. The UK Collaborative Study has shown that the optimum time for measurement of serum AFP is between 16 and 18 weeks of pregnancy (Figure 14.3). At this time the detection efficiencies for both anencephaly and spina bifida at the 95th percentile of the normal range are 88% (Table 14.5). Detection efficiencies decrease somewhat if higher percentiles of the normal range are chosen as the cut-off point. Although a 95th percentile of the

TABLE 14.5 Proportion of NTD where maternal serum AFP concentrations at 16–18 weeks were above defined percentiles of the normal range. Data abstracted from the UK Collaborative Study

| | Percentile of the normal range | | | | |
	95th	96th	97th	98th	99th
Anencephaly	88	88	86	84	84
Open spina bifida	88	82	76	76	70

TABLE 14.6 Relationship between screening percentile and number of amniocenteses performed. Data from Edinburgh screening trial

Samples assayed (15–21 weeks)	9705
Raised AFP value on first sample	602 (6.2%)
Raised AFP value on first and second sample	370 (3.8%)
Underestimated gestation	77
Twins observed on ultrasonic scan	18
Threatened or missed abortion	26
Amniocentesis declined	19
Amniocentesis carried out	230 (2.4%)

normal range as initial cut-off implies that up to 5% of pregnancies may be subjected to amniocentesis, the actual number of amniocenteses performed is usually much less. Thus our own experience in Edinburgh (Table 14.6) shows that even when the 94th percentile was used as the primary cut-off, only 2.5% of pregnancies were actually subjected to amniocentesis[15].

14.3.3 Other abnormalities associated with elevated maternal serum AFP

A number of other abnormalities have been reported to be associated with elevations of maternal serum AFP. These include most fetal defects where the amniotic fluid is increased, such as intrauterine death, congenital nephrosis, exomphalos, duodenal and oesophageal atresias, and Meckel syndrome. It seems reasonable to conclude that if the amniotic fluid AFP is strongly increased this will be reflected in a concomitant increase in maternal serum AFP[16].

However, maternal serum AFP may sometimes be raised in the absence of an amniotic fluid AFP increase. The most common situation where this occurs is threatened abortion. In one sense this raises a problem in that amniocentesis is strongly contraindicated if there is a likelihood of the patient miscarrying. The question then arises as to whether the increase in serum AFP is signalling an impending abortion (where amniocentesis should be avoided) or an open neural tube defect (where amniocentesis should be performed for diagnostic purposes). This dilemma has been resolved by the observation that serum AFP values in threatened abortion are only increased when there are overt clinical signs of vaginal bleeding[17]. When bleeding is present it is recommended that amniocentesis be delayed until the pregnancy 'settles' or the problem is resolved by miscarriage.

14.3.4 Multiple pregnancy

In multiple pregnancy maternal serum AFP is somewhat increased. The UK Collaborative Study showed that approximately 30% of twin pregnancies would be revealed by AFP values above the 95th percentile of the normal range (Table 14.7). It has been shown that the median serum AFP value is approximately doubled in twin pregnancy and trebled in a triplet pregnancy[18,19]. Thus each fetus appears to contribute actively to the level of AFP in maternal serum.

TABLE 14.7 Proportion of twin pregnancies where maternal serum AFP concentrations were above defined percentiles of the normal range. Data abstracted from the UK Collaborative Study

| Gestation in weeks | Percentile of normal range for singletons | | |
	95th	97th	99th
13–15	31	25	12
16–18	34	23	17
19–21	36	32	27

14.3.5 Future prospects

The value of maternal serum AFP screening for fetal neural tube defects has now been well established. One exciting new development which has arisen directly from a screening programme is the discovery of a significant association between elevated maternal serum AFP and the eventual delivery of an infant with low birth-weight[20,21]. The premature infant, whether of low birth-weight, short gestation or both, is a major factor in the continuing high rates of perinatal and infant mortality in developed countries. Though the association between low birth-weight and serum AFP is a statistically significant one (Table 14.8), it is not at present a practical aid to the management of these high risk pregnancies. However, it must be noted that measurements of AFP were made between 15 and 20 weeks of pregnancy, which has been shown to be optimum for the detection of anencephaly and spina bifida. It seems possible that if measurements of serum AFP are made throughout pregnancy the detection rate for infants of inappropriate birth-weight may be increased to a point where AFP becomes a significant factor in the management of these pregnancies. While the last five years have seen enormous improvements in our ability to diagnose neural tube defects, we hope the next five years will see equally significant achievements in our ability to predict and eventually to prevent the birth of premature infants.

TABLE 14.8   Relationship between elevated maternal serum AFP at 15–20 weeks and infants of low birth-weight

Number with elevated maternal serum AFP	103
Outcome twins, spontaneous abortion or NTD	28 (27.2%)
Outcome singleton with birth-weight less than 2.5 kg	11 (10.7%)*
Outcome singleton with birth-weight greater than 2.5 kg	64 (62.1%)

*In the population as a whole, birth-weights of less than 2.5 kg represent 4.0% of the total.

References

1. Bergstrand, C. G. and Czar, B. (1956). Demonstration of a new protein fraction in serum from the human fetus. *Scand. J. Clin. Lab. Invest.*, **8**, 174
2. Brock, D. J. H. (1974). The molecular nature of alphafetoprotein in anencephaly and spina bifida. *Clin. Chim. Acta*, **57**, 315
3. Brock, D. J. H. and Sutcliffe, R. G. (1972). Alphafetoprotein in the antenatal diagnosis of anencephaly and spina bifida. *Lancet*, **ii**, 197
4. Brock, D. J. H. and Scrimgeour, J. B. (1972). Early prenatal diagnosis of anencephaly. *Lancet*, **ii**, 1252

5. Brock, D. J. H., Scrimgeour, J. B. and Nelson, M. M. (1975). Amniotic fluid alphafetoprotein measurements in the early diagnosis of central nervous system disorders. *Clin. Genet.*, **7**, 163

6. Brock, D. J. H. (1977). In *Progress in Medical Genetics*. New Series, Vol. 2, pp. 1–37

7. Brock, D. J. H. (1975). Antenatal misdiagnosis of neural tube defects. *Lancet,* **ii**, 495

8. Brock, D. J. H. and Gosden, C. M. (1977). Are second trimester amniotic fluids being properly examined? *Lancet*, **ii**, 1168

9. Brock, D. J. H. (1976). Prenatal diagnosis–chemical methods. *Br. Med. Bull.*, **32**, 16

10. Chemke, J., Miskin, A., Rau-Acha, Z., Porath, A., Sagir, M. and Katz, Z. (1977). *Clin. Genet.*, **ii**, 285

11. Brock, D. J. H., Bolton, A. E. and Monaghan, J. M. (1973). Prenatal diagnosis of anencephaly through maternal serum alphafetoprotein measurement. *Lancet,* **ii**, 923

12. Brock, D. J. H., Bolton, A. E. and Scrimgeour, J. B. (1974). Prenatal diagnosis of spina bifida and anencephaly through maternal plasma-alphafetoprotein measurement. *Lancet,* **i**, 767

13. Brock, D. J. H., Scrimgeour, J. B., Bolton, A. E., Wald, N. J., Peto, R. and Barker, S. (1975). Affect of gestational age on screening for neural defects by maternal plasma-AFP measurement. *Lancet,* **ii**, 195

14. Report of UK Collaborative Study on alpha-fetoprotein in relation to neural tube defects (1977). *Lancet*, **i**, 1323

15. Brock, D. J. H., Scrimgeour, J. B., Stephen, D., Barron, L. and Watt, M. (1978). Maternal plasma alphafetoprotein screening for fetal neural tube defects. *Br. J. Obstet. Gynaecol.* (In press)

16. Brock, D. J. H. (1976). The prenatal diagnosis of neural tube defects. *Obstet. Gynaecol. Survey*, **31**, 32

17. Wald, N. J., Barker, S., Cuckle, H., Brock, D. J. H. and Stirratt, G. M. (1976). Maternal serum AFP and spontaneous abortion. *Br. J. Obstet. Gynaecol.*, **84**, 357

18. Garoff, L. and Seppala, M. (1975). Alphafetoprotein and human placental lactogen levels in maternal serum in multiple pregnancies. *J. Obstet. Gynaecol. Br. Commonw.*, **80**, 695

19. Wald, N., Barker, S., Peto, R., Brock, D. J. H. and Bonnar, J. (1975). Maternal serum alphafetoprotein levels in multiple pregnancy. *Br. Med. J.*, **1**, 651

20. Wald, N., Cuckle, H., Stirratt, G. M., Bennett, M. J. and Turnbull, A. C. (1977). Maternal serum alphafetoprotein and low birth-weight. *Lancet*, **ii**, 268

21. Brock, D. J. H., Barron, L., Jelen, P., Watt, M. and Scrimgeour, J. B. (1977). Maternal serum alphafetoprotein measurements as an early indicator of low birth-weight. *Lancet*, **ii**, 267

15

Alphafetoprotein in oncology
J. Kohn

15.1	INTRODUCTION	177
15.2	HEPATOCELLULAR CARCINOMA	178
	15.2.1 Incidence of AFP positivity	178
	15.2.2 Differential diagnosis of AFP elevations	179
15.3	ABDOMINAL TUMOURS IN CHILDHOOD	179
	15.3.1 Non-neoplastic causes of elevated AFP in childhood	180
15.4	GERM CELL TUMOURS	180
15.5	CONCLUSIONS	182

15.1 INTRODUCTION

Alphafetoprotein (AFP), along with Bence Jones protein, βHCG and possibly thyrocalcitonin, is one of the few tumour related antigens that can be used successfully both in diagnosis and monitoring of neoplasia. The specificity of AFP as a tumour marker, particularly with respect to the germ cell tumours, is quite impressive. Although AFP can be used with considerable benefit as a diagnostic marker, its real value lies in the management of disease and in prognosis.

To be of clinical value, a tumour marker must fulfil certain requirements: it must be specific, sensitive and be reasonably simple to assay. Ideally, it should also provide a lead time in those cases that are potentially treatable. The accumulated experience over the last 15 years has shown that AFP fulfils all these criteria especially with respect to the germ cell tumours.

15.2 HEPATOCELLULAR CARCINOMA

The first demonstration of raised levels of AFP in association with neoplasia was by Abelev[1] in hepatocellular carcinoma experimental animals and by Taratinov[2] in human subjects. AFP production by hepatocellular carcinoma can easily be demonstrated by immunofluorescent staining of animal tumours but proves more difficult in human tumours, probably because of the very rapid synthesis and release of AFP from the cell.

15.2.1 Incidence of AFP positivity

One of the fundamental requirements for a satisfactory tumour marker is sensitivity: the higher the incidence of positive results the better the marker. Unfortunately there has been considerable divergence of opinion on the sensitivity of AFP as a marker for hepatocellular carcinoma, particularly in the early reports, with the percentage positivity ranging from 38% to better than 90%[3]. Much of this divergence can be attributed to a failure of early authors to state their methods of detection and to the use of relatively insensitive immunodiffusion techniques. Over recent years there has been a gradual change to the more sensitive qualitative assays, radioimmunoassay and enzyme immunoassay, with consequent increase in positivity of the test.

In one early series from my own laboratory[4] we detected 84% of proven cases of hepatocellular carcinoma using a countercurrent electrophoresis technique with a lower limit of sensitivity of 200 μg/l. In a parallel series of 2118 cases known not to be hepatocellular carcinoma there were 39 positive results: 9 metastatic liver disease, 16 active cirrhosis and 14 undiagnosed. Many authors have suggested that there is a higher incidence of AFP positivity in non-Caucasians than in Caucasians[3]. This remains a controversial question although our own data shows no evidence of racial or sex difference in either AFP positivity or quantitative levels.

A simple qualitative screening technique such as this is not really good enough for monitoring the progress of a patient on treatment. The introduction of a radioimmunoassay for AFP soon showed that a proportion of proven hepatocellular carcinomas – probably not more than 6% – had levels below 200 μg/l but above the normal level which we arbitrarily set at 25 μg/l.

15.2.2 Differential diagnosis of AFP elevations

Various liver diseases, hepatitis, cirrhosis, acute liver failure, and metastatic liver disease may be associated with elevated AFP levels and give 'false positive' results on the screening test. Pregnancy is also associated with elevated AFP levels but this should not provide a diagnostic problem.

Cirrhosis and hepatitis present the most serious problems in the differential diagnosis of raised AFP levels, in that both may have similar clinical features and symptomatology to those of hepatocellular carcinoma. Here the repeat assay after an interval is of great value: in malignancy the level will rise whilst in cirrhosis and hepatitis the level will fluctuate and eventually fall. Serial measurement of AFP can be used as a prognostic indicator in acute liver failure following acute hepatitis or poisoning with such compounds as carbon tetrachloride or paracetamol.

15.3 ABDOMINAL TUMOURS IN CHILDHOOD

AFP is universally elevated in hepatoblastoma, levels usually reaching the mg/l range. The value of AFP in the differential diagnosis of abdominal tumours in childhood can be seen in Table 15.1.

TABLE 15.1 AFP screening in various tumours in childhood

		AFP screening test	
	n	Positive	Negative
Hepatoblastoma	45	45	0
Nephroblastoma	43	0	43
Neuroblastoma	42	0	42
Lymphoma	17	0	17
Osteosarcoma	19	0	19

15.3.1   Non-neoplastic causes of elevated AFP in childhood

AFP is elevated in ataxia telangiectasia[6] and in tyrosinosis[7]. Elevations have been reported in cystic fibrosis[8] but subsequent studies have tended to refute this observation[9,10]. In the neonatal period AFP levels are higher in hepatitis than in biliary atresia[11], a feature which may be of value in the differential diagnosis of neonatal jaundice.

15.4   GERM CELL TUMOURS

Both in diagnosis and in management of germ cell tumours AFP has proved to be of considerable value to the clinician. The diagnostic element may be rather less important in the testicular tumours in that the orchidectomy specimen will be available for histological examination, but an elevated AFP may signal the presence of teratomatous elements that have been overlooked on first histological examination.

AFP production by germ cell tumours is associated with the yolk sac elements in the tumour[12]. Trophoblastic or carcinomatous elements do not produce AFP. It follows from this that only a proportion of testicular teratomas can be expected to be associated with elevated AFP levels. The incidence of positivity is in the order of 65% when serial samples are analysed.

Seminomas are AFP negative. There have been isolated reports of AFP production by seminoma but in the majority of cases where there has been the opportunity, second look histology has revealed a combined tumour with teratomatous elements[12].

The real value of AFP in the management of germ cell tumours lies in the use of sequential samples to monitor therapy. The importance of sequential sampling techniques can be seen from two series of cases, one series in which

TABLE 15.2   Mortality in testicular teratoma in relation to post-orchidectomy AFP levels

Operative stage	AFP negative	AFP positive
I	2%	50%
II	8%	63%
III and IV	67%	86%

sequential samples were studied with a 65% AFP positivity, and a second series of random samples which showed only 30% positivity.

Sequential samples post-orchidectomy can be used as a guide to operative removal of the tumour; i.e. if after taking into account the 5 days half-life of AFP, the AFP remains elevated, or falls at a rate slower than would be expected from the half-life, then residual or metastatic tumour is present. The persistence of elevated AFP levels is correlated with poor prognosis[14] (Table 15.2).

Figure 15.1 illustrates the sequential AFP values in two patients, one with an apparent half-life (AHL) of 5 days and survival in excess of three years, and the other in whom there has been clinical recurrence. AHL is calculated from the formula shown in Figure 15.2. The retrospective application of this approach to 44 patients has shown that, of 35 with an AHL greater than 7 days 28 have died, whilst of 9 with an AHL of 5 days or less only one has died.

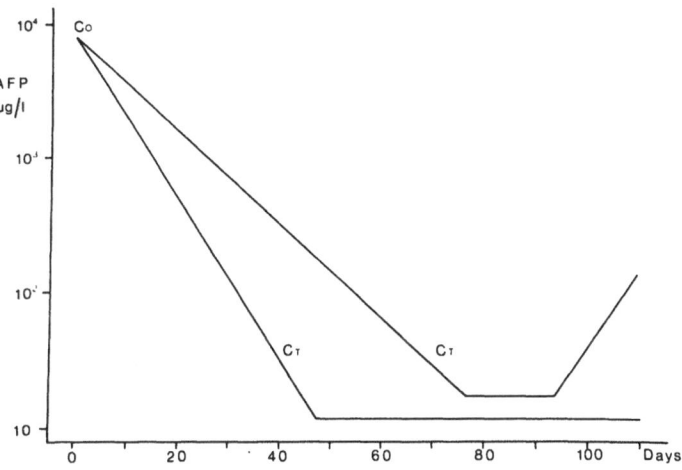

Figure 15.1   The apparent half-life (AHL) concept

$$\text{AHL} \;=\; \frac{-\,0.3 \times T}{\log^{10}\!\left(\dfrac{C_T}{C_O}\right)}$$

Figure 15.2   Calculation of AHL. T = time interval in days; C_O = initial AFP concentration (μg/l); C_T = AFP concentration (μg/l) after T days

15.5 CONCLUSIONS

AFP, assayed by a sensitive radioimmunoassay, is a valuable adjunct in the treatment and management of germ cell tumours and primary hepatic malignancy. The levels provide prognostic as well as diagnostic indications.

The sensitive, but qualitative, countercurrent immunoelectrophoretic technique is a useful technique for screening large numbers of patients with liver disease in the exclusion of hepatocellular carcinoma.

References

1. Abelev, G. I., Perova, S., Khramkova, N. L., Postnikova, Z. A. and Irlin, I. (1963). Production of embryonal alphaglobulin by the transplantable mouse hepatomas. *Transplant. Bull.*, **1**, 174
2. Taratinov, Y. S. (1964). Detection of embryospecific alphaglobulin in the blood sera of patients with primary liver tumour. *Vopr. Med. Khim.*, **10**, 90
3. Abelev, G. I. (1971). Alpha fetoprotein in ontogenesis and its association with malignant tumours. *Adv. Cancer Res.*, **14**, 295
4. Kohn, J. and Weaver, P. C. (1974). Serum alpha fetoprotein in hepatocellular carcinoma. *Lancet*, **ii**, 334
5. Kohn, J. (1973). Counter immunoelectrophoresis technique for the detection and identification of alpha fetoprotein. *Tumour Res.*, **8**, 42
6. Waldmann, T. A. and McIntire, K. R. (1972). Serum alpha fetoprotein levels in patients with ataxia telangiectasia. *Lancet*, **ii**, 1112
7. Belanger, L. (1973). Tyrosinémie héréditaire et alphafetoproteinie. *Pathol. Biol.*, **21**, 457
8. Chandra, R. K., Madhavankutty, K. and Way, R. C. (1975). Serum alpha fetoprotein in patients with cystic fibrosis and their parents and siblings. *Br. Med. J.*, **1**, 714
9. Wallwork, J. C., McFarlane, H., Hingley, S. and Milford Ward, A. (1975). Serum alpha fetoprotein in cystic fibrosis. *Br. Med. J.*, **2**, 392
10. Brock, D. J. H., Barron, L., Manson, J. and McCrae, W. M. (1978). Serum alpha fetoprotein in cystic fibrosis of the pancreas. *Clin. Chim. Acta*, **82**, 101
11. Zeltzer, P. M., Neerhout, R. C., Fonkalsrud, E. W. and Stiehm, E. R. (1974). Differentiation between neonatal hepatitis and biliary atresia by measuring serum alpha fetoprotein. *Lancet*, **i**, 373
12. Talerman, A. and Haije, W. G. (1974). Alpha fetoprotein and germ cell tumours: a possible role of yolk sac tumour in production of alpha fetoprotein. *Cancer*, **34**, 1722
13. Kohn, J., Orr, A. H., McElwain, T. J., Bentall, M. and Peckham, M. J. (1976). Serum alpha fetoprotein in patients with testicular tumours. *Lancet*, **ii**, 433
14. Kohn, J. (1976). Alpha fetoprotein in testicular tumours. In: *Oncodevelopmental Gene Expression*. p. 387. (New York: Academic Press)

16

α_1-Antitrypsin
A. Milford Ward

16.1 INTRODUCTION   185

16.2 GENETIC VARIATION   185
    16.2.1 *Anthropogenetics*   187
    16.2.2 *Inheritance*   188

16.3 QUANTITATION   189
    16.3.1 *Genetic influence on $\alpha_1 AT$ synthesis*   189
    16.3.2 *Reduced levels in disease*   190
    16.3.3 *Increased levels in disease*   190
    16.3.4 *Influence of drug therapy on $\alpha_1 AT$*   190

16.4 α_1AT GENETICS AND DISEASE ASSOCIATIONS   190
    16.4.1 *$\alpha_1 AT$ and lung disease*   191
    16.4.2 *$\alpha_1 AT$ and liver disease*   191
    16.4.3 *$\alpha_1 AT$ and rheumatic disease*   193
    16.4.4 *$\alpha_1 AT$ and renal disease*   193
    16.4.5 *$\alpha_1 AT$ and pregnancy*   193

16.5 CONCLUSION   194

TABLE 16.1 Protease inhibitors of human plasma

Protein	Abbreviation	M.wt. (daltons)	Mean concentration (g/l)	Molar concentration (μmol/l)	Enzymes inhibited in vivo
α_1-Antitrypsin	α_1AT	55000	2.0	36	Serine protease
α_1-Antichymotrypsin	α_1ACT	69000	0.4	7	?
α_1-Antithrombin (Antithrombin III)	AT III	65000	0.3	4.5	Thrombin
Inter α-trypsin inhibitor	1αTI	160000	0.4	3	?
α_2-Macroglobulin	α_2M	725000	2.0	2.7	Endoprotease, plasmin
α-Neuraminoglycoprotein (C1 inhibitor)	C1 INH	104000	0.25	2.5	C1s Activated Hageman factor

1.1 INTRODUCTION

α_1-Antitrypsin (α_1AT) is the major natural inhibitor of serine proteases of human plasma (Table 16.1), comprising some 90% of the total plasma tryptic inhibitory capacity. α_1AT is somewhat of a misnomer in that the protein has little chance to meet the secretory enzyme trypsin *in vivo* and exerts a wide spectrum of inhibition of proteolytic activity, exerting active inhibition of elastase, collagenase, thrombin, plasmin, renin, kallikrein and sperm acrosine, as well as bacterial and granulocyte proteases. α_1AT is a glycoprotein, molecular weight 50 000–55 000 daltons, containing 12.5% carbohydrate, and comprises about 75% of the α_1-globulin fraction. It is synthesized in the hepatic parenchymal cells and distributed throughout the intravascular and extravascular pool; as an acute phase reactant protein, the plasma level increases markedly as a result of trauma or infection.

First isolated by Schultze *et al.*[1], clinical interest in α_1AT was initiated by the description of a familial emphysema by Laurell and Eriksson in 1963[2].

16.2 GENETIC VARIATION

The initial description of a familial deficiency was rapidly superseded by the description of multiple genetic polymorphism[3]. The descriptions were refined by Fagerhol[4] under the name of the Pi system, Pi referring to protease inhibitor, and some 24 distinct types and subtypes are now recognized. The various alleles may be distinguished by discontinuous acid starch gel electrophoresis at pH 4.95[3], acid starch gel electrophoresis and crossed immunoelectrophoresis[5] and by isoelectric focusing in polyacrylamide gel[6] (Figure 16.1). The complete identification of all alleles also requires extended agarose electrophoresis at pH 8.6 and immunochemical quantitation of α_1AT[7]. There is good agreement in phenotype identification between the major techniques of acid starch gel electrophoresis and isoelectric focusing[8].

The most common allele in all population groups is designated Pi M, the other alleles having an alphabetic nomenclature which denotes their electrophoretic mobility relative to the 'normal' allele: Pi F being fast, Pi S slow and Pi Z very slow. The 24 alleles currently described are: B, C, D, E, E_2, F, G, I, L, M, M_2, M_3, M^Malton, N, P, S, V, W, W_2, X, Y, Y_2, Z and null. The null allele (Pi$^-$) is the allele of complete deficiency and can only be detected in its heterozygous state by family studies.

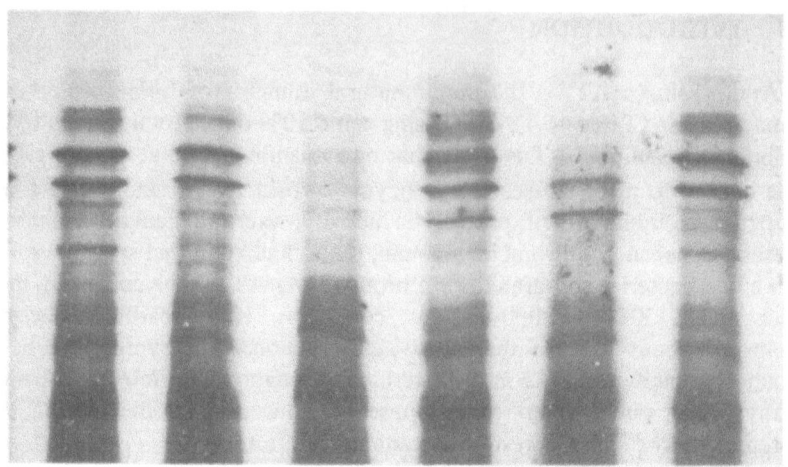

Figure 16.1 Pi phenotypes demonstrated by isoelectric focusing in thin layer poly-acrylamide gel with a pH gradient 4–5. (Anode at top). Left to right: Pi M, MZ, Z, MS, S, M

TABLE 16.2 Pi gene frequencies in various European populations

	Pi M	*Pi S*	*Pi Z*	*Pi F*
Sweden	0.945	0.027	0.024	0.003
UK (white)	0.897	0.050	0.017	0.030
Norway	0.946	0.023	0.016	0.013
Greece	0.959	0.003	0.016	0.013
Hungary	0.892	0.017	0.015	0.070
Spain	0.866	0.112	0.012	0.003
Germany	0.879	0.021	0.009	0.090
France	0.911	0.079	0.006	0.001
Portugal	0.859	0.115	0.018	

16.2.1 Anthropogenetics

The distribution of Pi phenotypes in different populations varies widely. Pi M in the homozygous form is the commonest phenotype in all populations studied. In Europe Pi F allele shows its highest frequency in Hungary and across the north German plain, whilst the Pi Z allele is commonest in Sweden and the Pi S allele in the Iberian peninsula (Table 16.2). Intermediate frequencies reflect population movements during history and the relatively high frequency of the Pi S allele in northern England may reflect the heavy commitment of Spanish troops in that area during the years of Roman occupation.

In the UK Caucasian population, just four alleles constitute more than 99% of the gene population: M 89.7%, S 5%, Z 1.7%; all other alleles having a frequency of 0.1% or less (Table 16.3).

TABLE 16.3 Incidence of various Pi phenotypes in a
UK Caucasian population

	%
Pi M	80.5
Pi MS	9.0
Pi FM	5.0
Pi MZ	3.0
Pi FS	0.30
Pi S	0.25
Pi SZ	0.17
Pi FZ	0.10
Pi F	0.09
Pi Z	0.03

All other phenotypes have a frequency of 0.01% or less

16.2.2   Inheritance

The alleles of the Pi system are inherited in mendelian fashion as codominant alleles acting at a single autosomal locus, although the precise chromosomal location of that locus has not been defined. The result of this codominant mendelian pattern of inheritance can be seen in family studies (Figure 16.2).

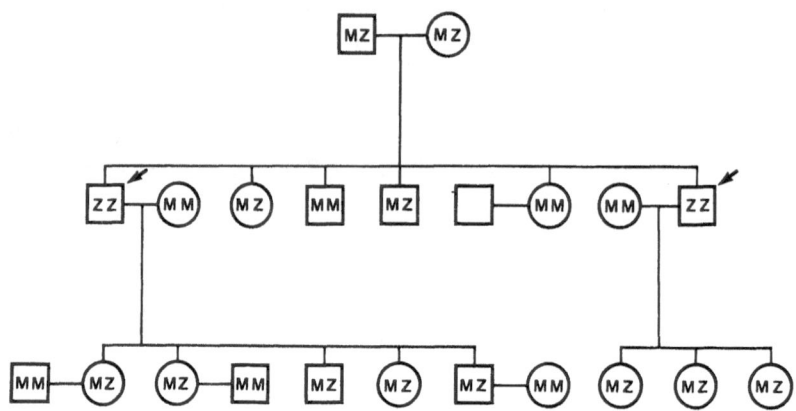

Figure 16.2   Inheritance of the Pi alleles: family study showing two Pi Z individuals, one of whom had severe lower lobe emphysema and the other micronodular cirrhosis

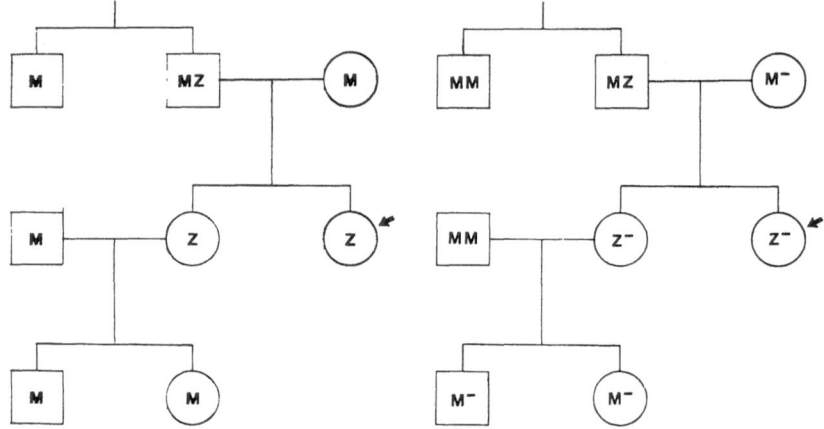

Figure 16.3   Inheritance of the Pi alleles: (a) anomalous inheritance pattern as defined prior to quantitation of α_1 AT and full phenotype evaluation, (b) inclusion of the null allele (Pi$^-$)

Because the phenotyping methods do not demonstrate the presence of the null allele, the apparent homozygote is conventionally reported as a single gene product, i.e. Pi M, unless family studies show the inheritance of Pi M alleles from both parents. The effect of the null allele on the apparent legitimacy of a family can be seen in Figure 16.3. Figure 16.3a shows the phenotypes as defined on initial testing, with inconsistencies in the mode of inheritance in the second and third generations; subsequent quantitative studies revealed half the expected α_1AT in certain family members and allowed the inclusion of the null allele as in Figure 16.3b.

16.3 QUANTITATION

α_1AT can be determined as plasma tryptic inhibitory capacity using benzoyl-arginine-p-nitroanilide as substrate[9] or immunochemically by single radial immunodiffusion, electroimmunodiffusion, automated immunoprecipitation or laser nephelometry.

Normal mean plasma level in adult Caucasians is 2.1 g/l with a standard deviation of 0.3 g/l. Levels in the newborn fully mature infant are similar to the adult but somewhat lower values are seen during the first 6 months of life.

16.3.1 Genetic influence on α_1AT synthesis

Most of the Pi alleles induce the same α_1AT synthesis, each allele acting independently. Low values reflect the lower rate of synthesis of certain alleles. The alleles responsible for reduced α_1AT synthesis and low plasma levels are: Pi W 80%, Pi S 60%, Pi P 25%, Pi Z 15% and Pi null 0%. Normal mean plasma levels of the Pi ZZ and Pi SS homozygotes are 15% and 60% respectively and of the Pi MZ and Pi MS heterozygotes 57.5% and 80% respectively of the normal mean value dominated by Pi MM (Table 16.4).

16.3.2 Reduced levels in disease

Low levels of α_1AT independent of genetic variants are seen in the neonatal respiratory distress syndrome[10]. Low levels are also seen as secondary features in association with renal or gastrointestinal protein-losing states. Low levels in jaundice herald the onset of acute yellow atrophy[11].

16.3.3 Increased levels in disease

α_1AT is an acute phase reactant protein and plasma levels rise in most acute inflammatory conditions and in cases of tissue necrosis. Elevations are much less marked in chronic inflammatory diseases and in collagen vascular diseases, rheumatoid arthritis and polyarteritis nodosa. α_1AT levels are markedly increased in active hepatitis and liver cirrhosis when other acute phase reactants are usually normal[12]. α_1AT levels are also raised in most tumour-bearing patients, the highest levels being achieved in widely disseminated metastatic disease.

α_1AT rises after surgery and, in the absence of infection or continuing tissue necrosis, returns to normal levels in 10–12 days.

16.3.4   Influence of drug therapy on α_1AT

Plasma levels of α_1AT increase by 50–100% following administration of exogenous oestrogens either as therapeutic agents or as oral contraceptives. This increase has been attributed to a synthesis-enhancing effect of oestrogen[9]. This synthesis-enhancement effect is seen in all phenotypes to a similar degree, but the absolute effect will be less dramatic in the Pi SZ and Pi Z phenotypes[13].

16.4 α_1AT GENETICS AND DISEASE ASSOCIATIONS

The original descriptions of Laurell and Eriksson[2] and Sharp *et al.*[14] of the associations of the Pi Z state with lower lobe emphysema and progressive juvenile cirrhosis respectively have initiated considerable clinical interest in the genetic basis of disease. In some instances the lowered tryptic inhibitory capacity of α_1AT-deficient individuals can be incriminated in the pathogenesis of a disease process, but in other instances such associations are not so clear. In these cases one has to propose gene linkage with some other factor, as yet unidentified, which may predispose to the disease in question.

TABLE 16.4   Mean antitrypsin concentration for different Pi phenotypes

Phenotype	% Normal	Mean concentration (g/l)
M	100	2.0
MS, FS	80	1.6
MP	62.5	1.3
S	60	1.2
MZ, FZ	57.5	1.1
M⁻	50	1.0
SZ	37.5	0.8
Z	15	0.3

16.4.1 α_1AT and lung disease

The association of α_1AT deficiency with predominantly lower lobe emphysema of early onset was first described by Laurell and Eriksson[2]. The homozygous Pi Z and to a similar extent the heterozygous Pi SZ are associated with a progressive panacinar emphysema of early onset (20–30 years). The predilection for the basal zones is related to the reduced vascular perfusion and to macrophage accumulation. The reduced tryptic inhibitory capacity is thought to allow increased tissue damage following lysozomal protease regurgitation during phagocytosis. Elastic recoil is diminished early[15] suggesting proteolytic damage to elastic fibres. Extrinsic lung irritants such as smoking and industrial pollutants appear to aggravate the lesion in genetically susceptible individuals. Primary lower lobe emphysema of α_1AT deficiency is not typically associated with bronchitis or asthma and, unlike other forms of emphysema, affects males and females in equal proportion.

The risk of lung disease in the Pi MZ heterozygote has been a point of some contention. Whilst Welch et al.[16] claimed there to be no increased risk, Lieberman[17] showed there to be a modest increased risk. More recent data has shown that the Pi MZ individual carries an 8-fold greater risk of lower lobe emphysema but that the condition develops at a later age (40–50 years) (Table 16.5).

In the absence of mass screening and follow-up studies it is difficult to tell what proportion of the Pi ZZ population develops emphysema. Some estimate can, however, be made by comparing the numbers of Pi ZZ patients with emphysema with the expected number of Pi ZZ individuals in the general population. Examination of data derived in this way suggests that about 60% of the Pi ZZ individuals develop emphysema.

There is little data on the incidence of Pi phenotype anomalies in other forms of lung disease although Geddes et al.[18] have shown an increase in non-M phenotypes, principally Pi MZ, in patients with cryptogenic fibrosing alveolitis.

16.4.2 α_1AT and liver disease

A second major clinical manifestation of the homozygous Pi Z state is transient cholestatic jaundice in the newborn proceeding to progressive juvenile cirrhosis[14,19]. The causal relationship between the Pi Z allele and liver damage is not clear but the retention with the hepatocyte of large quantities of α_1AT may prove to be a metabolic embarrassment to the cell. Liver biopsies from Pi ZZ individuals show characteristic PAS protein diastase resistant granules

TABLE 16.5 Pi phenotypes in lung disease: data derived from 650 new patients attending Respiratory Medicine Clinics, Sheffield, 1976–77

	Pi phenotype (% incidence)							
	M	MS	FM	MZ	S	SZ	Z	Others
Emphysema—generalised	84	8.5	2	4	—	—	—	1.5
Emphysema—lower lobe	60.5	8.0	—	19.5	3	1.5	3	4.5
Emphysema—with chronic bronchitis	83	9.5	—	5.5	1	—	—	1
Bronchitis and asthma	83	11	1	3.5	1	—	—	0.5
Bronchiectasis	78	10	1	8	1	—	—	2
Bronchial carcinoma	85.5	5.5	5.5	3	—	—	—	0.5
Fibrosing alveolitis	73	12.5	—	10.5	2	—	—	2
Normal population	80.5	9	5	3	0.25	0.17	0.03	2.05

within the hepatic parenchymal cells which can be stained specifically with fluorochrome-conjugated antiserum to α_1AT. Ultrastructural studies show that these granules are α_1AT contained within dilated cysternae of the endoplasmic reticulum. The accumulation of α_1AT within the hepatocyte is thought to be brought about by normal synthesis and reduced membrane transport interrupting release from the hepatocyte. The lack of one sialic acid residue on the Pi Z allele product may account for this impaired membrane transport.

The reported incidence of neonatal liver disease in the Pi ZZ population varies between 10 and 20%. Sveger[20], in a population screening programme, identified 40 children of Pi ZZ, 4 of whom developed jaundice and cirrhosis; Ward[21], on the other hand, reported 10 Pi ZZ children with jaundice and cirrhosis from a population that should have yielded 48 Pi ZZ individuals. From the available data it would appear that α_1AT deficiency accounts for 10% of all cases of transient neonatal jaundice in infants in whom structural biliary anomalies, hepatic immaturity and blood group incompatibility can be excluded.

Post-necrotic cirrhosis in α_1AT deficiency in adults has also been described in association with Pi ZZ[22], Pi SZ[11], Pi FZ[23] and Pi PZ. There also appears to be an increased frequency of non-M phenotypes in patients with hepatocellular carcinoma[24] and an increased incidence of Pi MZ in haemachromatosis.

16.4.3 α_1AT and rheumatic disease

An increased frequency of non-M phenotypes, principally Pi MZ has been reported in patients with rheumatoid arthritis (RA) and associated fibrosing alveolitis or other severe pulmonary manifestation[18]. Phenotype distribution in uncomplicated RA is not abnormal[18,25]. Pi MZ has also been shown to have an increased frequency among children with juvenile RA[26].

16.4.4 α_1AT and renal disease

A few reports have detailed cases of progressive glomerulonephritis or mesangiocapillary glomerulonephritis occurring in children and young adults in association with Pi Z[27,28,29].

16.4.5 α_1AT and pregnancy

α_1AT rises under oestrogenic stimulation to reach 2 to 3 times normal levels in the last trimester. The fall to normality occurs within the first two weeks *post partum.* As α_1AT is an inhibitor of sperm acrosine, it has been proposed that a low α_1AT level may be associated with an increased fertility; a proposal supported by the finding of increased numbers of Pi variants in women with large families[30].

16.5 CONCLUSION

It is unlikely that we have yet reached the end of the catalogue of diseases associated with Pi phenotype anomalies, although the aetiological relationships are far from clear. Reduced tryptic inhibitory capacity of the Pi $\acute{Z}$ homozygote and the Pi MZ heterozygote will undoubtedly have a bearing on the amount of tissue damage produced by an inflammatory episode, but other associations are not so immediately apparent. The hypothesis of the Pi genes being linked to other genes, as yet undetermined, which code for particular disease states remains unproven.

References

1. Schultze, H. E., Göllner, I., Heide, K., Schonenberger, M. and Schwick, G. (1955). Zur kenntnis der α-Globuline des menschlichen Normal senims. *Z. Naturforsch. B.*, **106**, 463
2. Laurell, C. B. and Eriksson, S. (1963). The electrophoretic alpha₁globulin pattern of serum $\alpha_1$antitrypsin deficiency. *Scand. J. Clin. Lab. Invest.*, **15**, 132
3. Fagerhol, M. K. and Braend, M. (1965). Serum prealbumin polymorphism in man. *Science*, **149**, 986
4. Fagerhol, M. K. (1968). The Pi system: Genetic variety of serum $\alpha_1$antitrypsin. *Ser. Haematol.*, **1**, 153
5. Fagerhol, M. K. and Laurell, C. B. (1967). The polymorphism of 'prealbumins' and $\alpha_1$antitrypsin in human sera. *Clin. Chim. Acta*, **16**, 199
6. Lebas, J., Hayem, A. and Martin, J. P. (1974). Etudes des variants genétique de l'$\alpha_1$antitrypsine en immunoelectrofocalisation bidimensionelle. *C.R. Acad. Sci. Paris*, **278**, 2359
7. Fagerhol, M. K. (1975). Pi typing techniques. *Prot. Biol. Fluids*, **22**, 493
8. Ward, A. M., Pickering, J. D., Fagerhol, M. K. and Martin, J. P. (1977). Pi (antitrypsin) typing methods: a comparison of acid starch gel electrophoresis and isoelectric focusing. *Hum. Hered.*, **27**, 292
9. Fagerhol, M. K. and Laurell, C. B. (1970). The Pi system: inherited variants of $\alpha_1$antitrypsin. *Prog. Med. Genet.*, **7**, 96
10. Mathis, R. K., Freier, E. F., Hunt, C. E., Krivit, W. and Sharp, H. L. (1973). Alpha₁antitrypsin in the respiratory distress syndrome. *N. Engl. J. Med.*, **288**, 59
11. Campra, J. L., Craig, J. R., Peters, R. L. and Reynolds, T. B. (1973). Cirrhosis associated with partial deficiency of $\alpha_1$antitrypsin in an adult. *Ann. Intern. Med.*, **78**, 233

12. Kindmark, C. O. and Laurell, C. B. (1972). Sequential changes of the plasma protein pattern in inoculation hepatitis. *Scand. J. Clin. Lab. Invest.*, **29**, Suppl. 124, 105

13. Lieberman, J. and Mittman, C. (1973). Dynamic response of alpha₁antitrypsin variants to diethyl stilboestrol. *Am. J. Human Genet.*, **25**, 610

14. Sharp, H. L., Bridges, R. A., Krivit, W. and Freier, E. F. (1969). Cirrhosis associated with $\alpha_1$antitrypsin deficiency: a previously unrecognised inherited disorder. *J. Lab. Clin. Med.*, **73**, 934

15. Kanner, R. E., Klauber, M. R., Watanabe, S. and Bigler, A. (1973). Pathologic patterns of obstructive pulmonary disease in patients with normal and deficient levels of $\alpha_1$antitrypsin. *Am. J. Med.*, **54**, 706

16. Welch, M. H., Reinecke, M. E., Hammerstein, J. F. and Fuenter, C. A. (1969). Antitrypsin deficiency in pulmonary disease: the significance of intermediate levels. *Ann. Intern. Med.*, **71**, 279

17. Lieberman, J. (1969). Heterozygous and homozygous $\alpha_1$antitrypsin deficiency in patients with pulmonary emphysema. *N. Eng. J. Med.*, **281**, 279

18. Geddes, D. M., Webley, M., Brewerton, D. A., Turton, C. W., Turner-Warwick, M., Murphy, A. H. and Ward, A. M. (1977). α_1Antitrypsin phenotypes in fibrosing alveolitis and rheumatoid arthritis. *Lancet,* **ii**, 1049

19. Ward, A. M. and Underwood, J. C. E. (1974). α_1Antitrypsin deficiency and liver disease in childhood: genetic immunochemical, histological and ultrastructural study, *J. Clin. Pathol.*, **27**, 467

20. Sveger, T. (1976). Liver disease in $\alpha_1$antitrypsin deficiency detected by screening of 200 000 infants. *N. Engl. J. Med.*, **294**, 1316   *Med.*,   **294**,   1316

21. Ward, A. M. (1975). α_1Antitrypsin (Pi) phenotypes in neonatal liver disease. *Prot. Biol. Fluids*, **22**, 521

22. Kumar, P., Lancaster Smith, M., Cook, P., Stansfeld, A., Clark, M. L. and Dawson, A. M. (1974). α_1Antitrypsin deficiency in chronic liver disease, and a report of cirrhosis and emphysema in adult members of a family. *Br. Med. J.*, **1**, 366

23. Brand, B., Bezahler, G. H. and Gould, R. (1974). Cirrhosis and heterozygous Pi FZ $\alpha_1$antitrypsin deficiency. *Gastroenterology,* **66**, 264

24. Berg, N. O. and Eriksson, S. (1972). Liver disease in adults with $\alpha_1$antitrypsin deficiency. *N. Engl. J. Med.*, **287**, 1264

25. Sjöblom, K. G. and Wollheim, F. A. (1977). α_1Antitrypsin phenotypes and rheumatic diseases. *Lancet,* **ii**, 41

26. Arnaud, P., Galbraith, R. M., Page Faulk, W. and Ansell, B. M. (1977). Increased frequency of the MZ phenotype of α_1 protease inhibitor in juvenile chronic polyarthritis. *J. Clin. Invest.*, **60**, 1442

27. Ward, A. M., Pickering, J. D. and Shortland, J. R. (1975). The renal manifestations of Pi Z. *Alpha₁antitrypsin and Pi system;* INSERM, 40, 131

28. Cox, D. W. (1974). Personal communication.

29. Miller, F. and Kuschner, M. (1969). α_1Antitrypsin deficiency, emphysema, necrotising angiitis and glomerulonephritis. *Am. J. Med.*, **46**, 615

30. Fagerhol, M. K. and Gedde Dahl, T. (1969). Genetics of the Pi serum types: family studies of the inherited variants of serum₁ α antitrypsin. *Hum. Hered.*, **19**, 354

17

Haptoglobin and orosomucoid in lung and breast tumours
A. R. Bradwell

17.1	INTRODUCTION	198
17.2	SERUM PROTEIN CHANGES IN PATIENTS WITH LUNG TUMOURS	198
	17.2.1 *Protein concentrations and tumour mass*	198
	17.2.1.1 *Patients, materials and methods*	198
	17.2.1.2 *Results*	199
	17.2.1.3 *Discussion*	201
	17.2.2 *Relationship of protein changes to prognosis*	201
	17.2.2.1 *Patients, materials and methods*	201
	17.2.2.2 *Results*	202
	17.2.2.3 *Discussion*	203
	17.2.3 *Monitoring of patients with lung cancer using serum proteins*	204
	17.2.3.1 *Patients, materials and methods*	204
	17.2.3.2 *Results*	206
	17.2.3.3 *Discussion*	207
17.3	SERUM PROTEIN CHANGES IN PATIENTS WITH BREAST TUMOURS	209
	17.3.1 *Introduction, materials and methods*	210
	17.3.2 *Results*	211
	17.3.2.1 *Haptoglobin*	211
	17.3.2.2 *Pregnancy-associated α_2-glycoprotein (PAG)*	212
	17.3.2.3 *Carcinoembryonic antigen (CEA)*	212
17.4	CONCLUSION	213

17.1 INTRODUCTION

With the improving efficacy of chemotherapeutic agents the early detection of recurrent disease in patients with neoplasia is becoming increasingly important. Available methods of detecting tumours are largely based on clinical and radiological techniques but these are generally insensitive. Recently there has been a search for more sensitive methods of tumour detection based upon serum measurements of tumour products. In particular carcino-embryonic antigen (CEA) has been shown to be useful in monitoring bowel and breast tumours while α-fetoprotein levels are useful for detecting and monitoring hepatomas[1-2].

Serum protein abnormalities also occur as a result of a host response to the growing tumour, and the serum concentration of many substances, including haptoglobin and orosomucoid, is increased in patients with carcinoma of the lung[3] and other tumours[4]. In this study we have attempted to evaluate the role of serum protein tests in patients with lung tumours and, to a lesser extent, breast tumours.

17.2 SERUM PROTEIN CHANGES IN PATIENTS WITH LUNG TUMOURS

Marked changes in the concentration of serum proteins in patients with lung tumours have been demonstrated[3]. The disease is common and patients usually have a short survival which allows easy assessment of any potential marker. This makes the tumour particularly suitable for study but staging is difficult and the benefits of a useful marker must be weighed against the present-day treatment which is far from satisfactory.

17.2.1 Protein concentrations and tumour mass

The concentration of any useful tumour marker must relate to the tumour mass. The mass of lung tumour can only be assessed at operation and at a stage before the tumour has widely metastasized. Any group of patients filling these criteria will therefore be highly selected.

17.2.1.1 *Patients, materials and methods*

Seventy-one patients who were attending a chemotherapy and immunotherapy clinic after radical resection of a primary lung tumour were studied[5]. The patients had been selected for the purposes of the trial on the following criteria:

(1) There was no macroscopic evidence of residual disease after the operation, as judged by the surgeon.

(2) The patients had a relatively poor prognosis on histological grounds (well-differentiated, keratinizing, squamous cell carcinomata were excluded).

(3) There was no clinical, radiological or scan evidence of residual metastatic disease.

The tumours in the resected lungs were examined macroscopically and histologically. The diameter of each tumour was measured in three dimensions and the mean calculated. Serum samples were collected prior to operation, stored at −20 °C and subsequently analysed for haptoglobin and orosomucoid using rocket immunoelectrophoresis[6] with a Hyland Standard serum (E3651 800B1) as the 100% reference value. Haptoglobin phenotypes were determined by polyacrylamide disc gel electrophoresis.

17.2.1.2   Results

There was a highly significant relationship between serum haptoglobin and orosomucoid concentrations and tumour diameter (Figure 17.1 and Table 17.1) (the numbers in each group are not identical because it was not possible to collect all the data on all the patients).

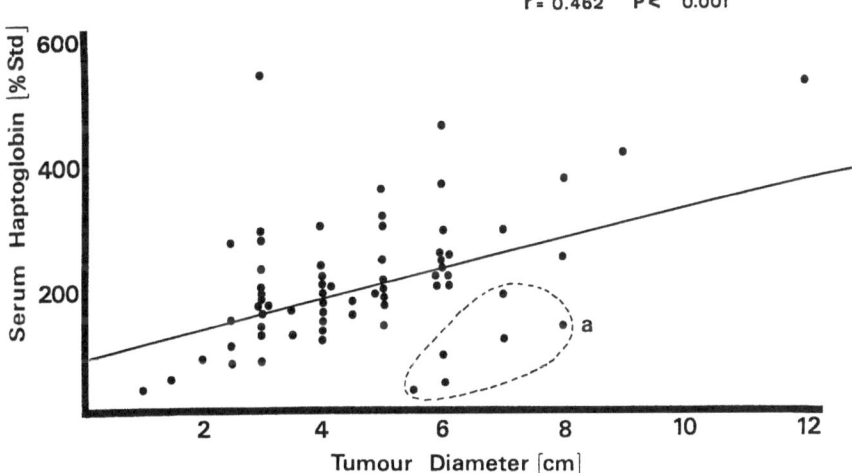

Figure 17.1   The relationship between pre-operative serum haptoglobin concentration and primary tumour diameter in patients with cancer of the lung. The patients comprising group (a) are those with low protein concentrations who had relatively long survival

TABLE 17.1 Relationship between the protein concentrations, tumour size and survival

	Haptoglobin (% standard)	Orosomucoid (% standard)	CRP (mg/l)	CEA (μg/l)	Survival (months)
Tumour diameter (cm)	0.462 $p<0.001$ (68)	0.394 $p<0.001$ (67)	0.317 $p<0.01$ (68)	0.159 NS (64)	0.122 NS (23)
Survival (months)	−0.401 NS (23)	−0.548 $p<0.01$ (22)	−0.392 NS (21)	−0.07 NS (23)	—
Survival for residual protein value	−0.689 $p<0.001$ (23)	−0.724 $p<0.001$ (22)	−0.455 $p<0.05$ (21)	0.051 NS (23)	—
Orosomucoid (% standard serum)	0.814 $p<0.001$ (71)	—	0.706 $p<0.001$ (68)	0.065 NS (67)	
CRP (mg/l)	0.684 $p<0.001$ (68)	—	—	−0.064 NS (67)	
CEA (μg/l)	0.135 NS (65)	—	—	—	

The statistical significance of each correlation coefficient (p) is given.
NS = not significant.
The numbers of patients are given in parenthesis.
For comparison with haptoglobin and orosomucoid the C-reactive protein (CRP) and carcinoembyronic antigen (CEA) serum concentrations measured in the same patients are also shown

Features that did not appear to influence protein concentrations were the degree of tumour necrosis, haemorrhage, inflammation in the lung and tumour histology and there was no significant correlation between tumour size and survival in this group of patients. There was no association between the concentrations of the haptoglobin genetic variants and tumour size.

17.2.1.3 Discussion

The results indicate that there is a highly significant relationship between tumour size and the serum concentrations of haptoglobin and orosomucoid in this highly selected group of patients. This relationship did not depend upon histological type or the presence or absence of metastases in the mediastinal lymph nodes. In addition the wide variation in pathological features resulting from the local effects of the tumour, such as lung necrosis, haemorrhage or localized pneumonia did not appear to adversely affect this relationship. This host response of the proteins did appear to depend upon the tumour size above all other parameters. Serum concentrations of proteins depend upon rates of production, distribution and catabolism, so no simple explanation of the results is possible, but it was curious that there was apparently a linear relationship between the two. One might have expected tumour mass or surface area to be more relevant.

In a further study of these patients no relationship was noted between CEA and tumour diameter. This is probably because CEA was elevated above 40 ng/l in only eight patients and its production by tumours is variable.

17.2.2 Relationship of protein changes to prognosis

Having established that tumour size relates to the serum protein concentrations, we then studied the relationship between the protein concentrations and the patients' survival time. All the patients had had their primary lung tumours resected and all had received chemotherapy. The effect this may have had on the patients' outcome is unknown but there is little evidence that surgical or medical intervention affects prognosis.

17.2.2.1 Patients, materials and methods

Twenty-three of the patients studied (17.2.1.1) died within 2 years of their operation. Their clinical details and serum protein concentrations were as before (17.2.1.1).

17.2.2.2   *Results*

The relationship between protein concentration and survival was significant for orosomucoid but was not significant for haptoglobin (Figure 17.2 and Table 17.1).

From Figure 17.1 it is apparent that many of the patients had protein concentrations considerably higher than the mean for a given tumour diameter and equally there was a group of patients (a) who had values of both proteins considerably lower than the mean (Figure 17.1). If the regression line of Figure 17.1 (for clarity this will be called the 'predicted protein values') represents the influence of the primary or measurable tumour upon the serum protein concentration, then the values above the regression line might be due to tumour elsewhere, i.e. undetected metastatic tumour. To determine whether this was the case, the predicted protein concentration was subtracted from the actual protein concentration to give a 'residual' value for each patient. The results were plotted against the time to death for each patient where this was known. Figure 17.3 shows there is now a highly significant relationship between the residual protein value and survival for haptoglobin. This relationship was also true for orosomucoid ($p < 0.001$). Patients who had protein concentrations greater than predicted died significantly earlier than patients with low protein concentrations. Furthermore, there was a small group of patients (Figure 17.3) who had markedly low protein concentrations and

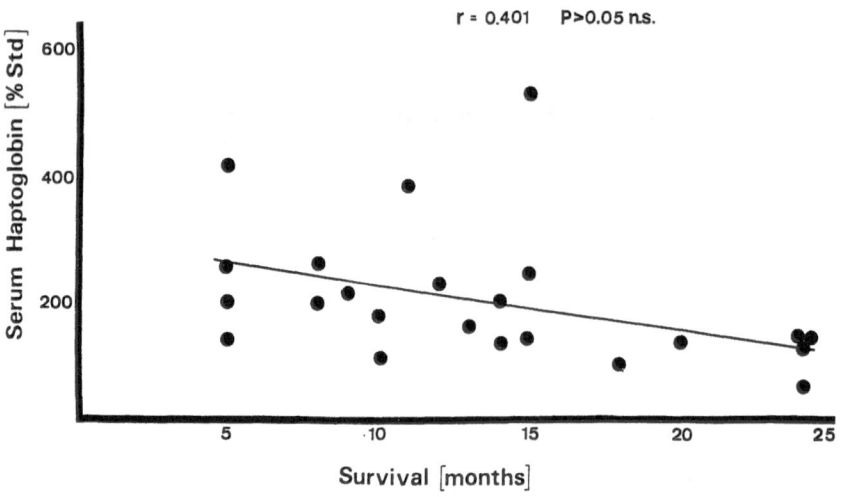

Figure 17.2   The relationship between pre-operative haptoglobin concentrations and survival time from operation in patients with cancer of the lung

survived for 24 months. Two of these patients had oatcell tumours with mediastinal lymph node involvement at the time of operation.

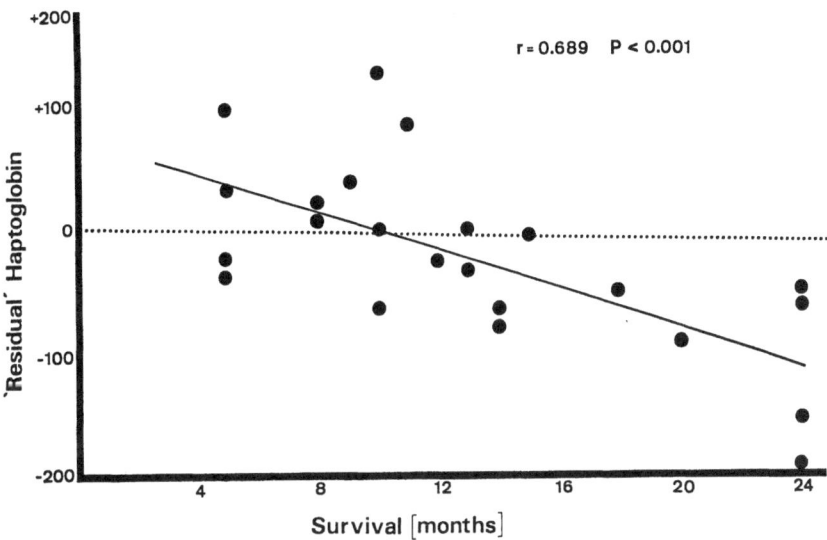

Figure 17.3 The relationship between 'residual' haptoglobin concentrations and survival times of patients

17.2.2.3   Discussion

There was, at best, only a poor relationship between the patients' survival and the 'uncorrected' protein concentrations (Figure 17.2). When the effect of the primary tumour was taken into account by calculating the residual protein value, a clear relationship between survival and this residual protein concentration existed. The shorter survival of patients with high residual values was probably due to unrecognized metastatic disease. Presumably such metastases were small as they were not detected by the normal clinical and radiological techniques. A positive residual protein concentration might be a useful measure of metastatic tumour at the time of operation.

Some patients had protein concentrations markedly lower than the predicted value for their respective tumour size and in some cases the values were actually less than the normal reference serum. As a group these patients had a favourable survival rate, in spite of unfavourable histology (including two patients with oatcell tumours and mediastinal lymph nodes containing microscopic tumour).

These low protein concentrations were consistent on repetition of the assays and, for haptoglobin, were not due to genetic variants. In addition, these patients had low C-reactive protein concentrations. A further feature of these patients was that the serum protein concentrations remained low even with the development of secondary disease[3]. Why such patients should have a favourable prognosis is unknown. However, prognosis was more accurately assessed by the patients' residual protein values than by conventional methods of assessing survival such as histological type or node involvement. A relationship between tumour size and prognosis after resection has been demonstrated[7] but was not apparent at a significant level in this study, perhaps because of the relatively small numbers involved.

17.2.3   Monitoring of patients with lung cancer using serum proteins

We have shown in section 17.2.1.2 that the serum concentrations of hapto-globin and orosomucoid are related to tumour size. This would imply that for any one patient the protein concentrations should rise during the progress of the disease. This has been assessed in the same patients who were attending the trial.

17.2.3.1   Patients, materials and methods

Thirty-seven of the patients who were attending the trial of chemotherapy and immunotherapy described above (17.2.1.1) were studied. The patients were assessed clinically and radiographically at the time of operation, at the time of chemotherapy (6 and 10 weeks after operation) and subsequently every three months, or more frequently, as clinically indicated. At each attendance blood samples were taken and the serum stored at $-20\,^{\circ}C$ to be analysed when convenient by the methods outlined above (17.2.1.1). The normal protein concentration ranges for these patients were based on a retrospective analysis of the serial protein concentrations and were chosen to keep false positives and false negatives to a minimum (see discussion 17.2.3.3). At the time of operation and at three-monthly intervals, or less if clinically indicated, radiological skeletal surveys and bone, brain and liver scans were performed.

TABLE 17.2 The numbers of months in advance of clinically detectable secondary disease that the proteins became significantly abnormal

Patient no.	Haptoglobin >150%	Orosomucoid >150%	CEA >40µg/l	CRP >20mg/l	ESR >40mm/h	Degree of change at death	Scans
2	5	5	8	12	0	*	
4	3	3	3	3	7	***	
5	6	5	7	6		***	2 Bone
6						0	
9	3	2			3	***	
10	0			3		*	0 Brain (P)
11	2					*	2 Liver (P)
12	3	3		3		***	0 Liver (P)
13	3	3		5	3	***	1 Liver (P)
14		3				***	
16	0					*	0 Bone (P)
17	5	5		5	5	**	
18	10	8		10	3	**	
19	0					*	0 Bone X-ray
22	3	3		3	3	**	
23	3	3	3	3	3	**	
29	3	3		3	3	***	3 Bone (P)
31	8	8	3	8	6	**	
34	3	3		3	3	***	0 X-ray
TOTAL 19	14	14	5	13	10		
Mean no. of months in advance	4.29	4.07	4.8	5.1	3.9		

A figure 0 indicates abnormality at the time of clinical metastases and a blank space shows where a test was abnormal only after secondary disease was clinically detected. Degree of change at the time of death indicated as *** large; ** moderate; * slight; 0 no change.

Scans—numbers indicate months in advance of clinical disease that scans became abnormal. (P) denotes probably positive scan

17.2.3.2   *Results*

The results of the measurement of haptoglobin and orosomucoid and three other parameters are shown in Table 17.2. This applies to the 19 patients who developed clinical metastases during the study.

The table shows that haptoglobin and orosomucoid provide almost equal information about tumour recurrence but are to some extent complementary. CEA was abnormal at an early stage in five patients, and ESR in ten patients. Table 17.2 shows that patients who had no protein changes before the clinical appearance of metastases tended to have little protein disturbance even at the time of death. Conversely the 'responders' showed progressive protein changes as the tumour bulk increased. There was no apparent relationship to the tumour histology or known organ involvement. Radiology including skeletal surveys and scans were at no time abnormal before the protein changes and were rarely abnormal before clinically evident disease.

Figure 17.4 shows the sequential protein changes in patient No. 6 during the development of secondary disease.

Three patients showed no significant protein changes during the increase in tumour size and neither did they show changes in the X-rays or scans.

Eighteen of the 37 patients did not develop overt clinical or radiological evidence of disease during the study and remained well. Eight of these patients have had increasing concentrations of haptoglobin and orosomucoid for one to eight months. The outcome of these patients is not known but the patterns of change are similar to those patients who subsequently developed clinical metastases. So far they show no X-ray or scan abnormalities. Seven of the 18 patients showed no significant changes in the proteins during the study. Two of the patients have shown small transient increases in haptoglobin and orosomucoid which did not coincide with known changes in the tumour status. Measurements of subsequent blood samples showed normal protein concentrations. Finally, one of the patients had a persistent marked increase in the proteins for nine months after chemotherapy with no apparent cause. He then developed a nephrotic syndrome possibly related to the therapy or the tumour. These latter three patients represent false positives.

Ten patients showed sequential reduction in their protein concentrations after chemotherapy (e.g. Figure 17.5, patient No. 9). Similar changes occurred in one patient after X-irradiation for superior vena cava obstruction. These changes appeared to be related to the changing tumour mass.

Four episodes of intercurrent illness were documented, such as severe bronchitis (Figure 17.4), coronary thrombosis, saphenofemoral bypass operation for peripheral vascular disease and deep venous thrombosis. The concentrations of the proteins were normal when measured three to six weeks after the illness and did not confuse the assessment of the patients' tumour status.

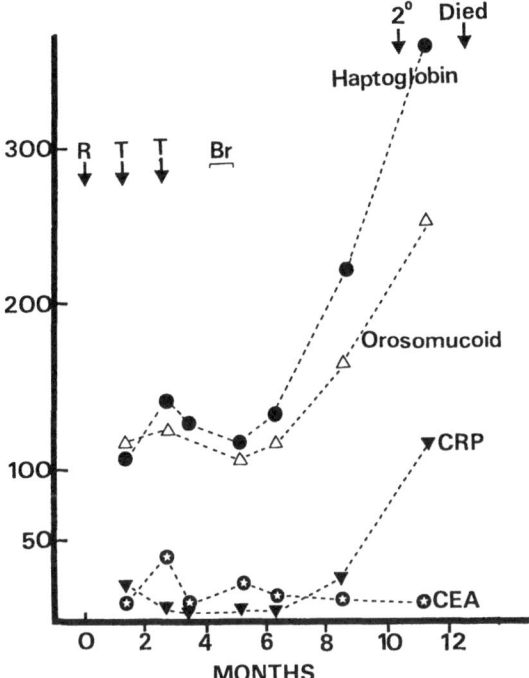

Figure 17.4 Serial measurements of haptoglobin, orosomucoid, CRP and CEA in a male patient who was followed-up until death. R=time of resection; T=chemotherapy; Br indicates a period of Bronchitis; 2° indicates where clinical secondaries were detected.
Haptoglobin and orosomucoid measured as % standard serum, CEA μg/l and CRP mg/l

17.2.3.3   Discussion

To be a useful marker for monitoring tumours, a test should ideally have the following characteristics:

(1) Concentrations should relate to the size and progress of the tumour.

(2) Changes should preferably be in advance of other methods of tumour detection.

(3) There should be a worthwhile number of positive results compared with false positives and false negatives.

(4) Treatment and drugs should not interfere with the tests.

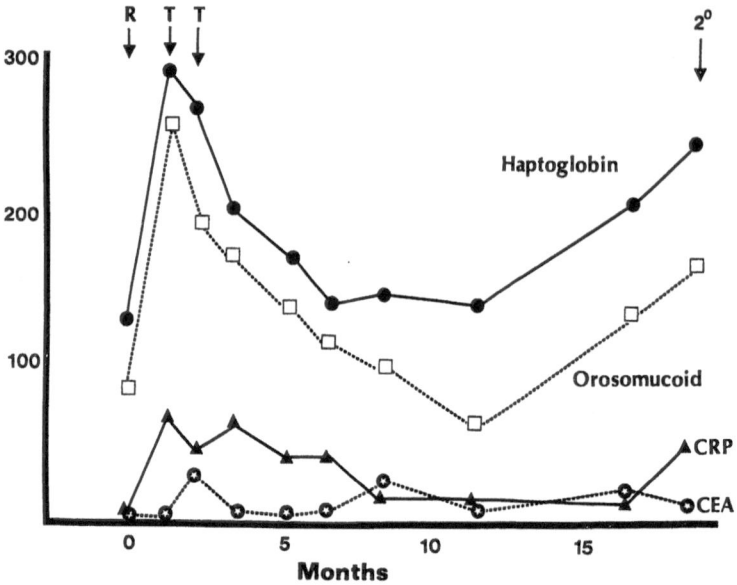

Figure 17.5 Protein measurements showing reduction of haptoglobin, CRP and orosomucoid concentrations following chemotherapy. For explanation of abbreviations, see Figure 17.4

(5) Non-specific influences, such as inflammation, should not interfere with the tests particularly when they cannot be identified.

(6) The test should indicate recurrent disease at a stage that is still treatable.

(7) It should be simple and cheap to perform.

Serum haptoglobin and orosomucoid measurements described here fit many of these criteria in patients with carcinoma of the lung. Both relate to the primary tumour size and to the increasing metastatic tumour mass, and the concentrations at the time of operation are of prognostic value. They provide early warning of tumour recurrence and are more reliable than diagnostic radiology or technetium scans, even though these methods have been advocated for detecting early recurrent disease.

Any diagnostic test should have a satisfactory number of positive results and a minimum of false positives and negative results. In the patients we studied the frequency of these could be selected depending upon the degree of protein abnormality one chose to indicate definite disease. The degree of changes that occurred as a result of metastatic tumour development was great enough in most patients to make this distinction relatively easy. However, by choosing these criteria for all the patients, some patients who developed metastatic disease were not regarded as having abnormal tests. These patients were those who tended to have a low normal protein level, and, in spite of doubling or trebling the protein concentrations during the development of metastases, the test was still below our criteria of abnormality. In some patients a percentage increase in concentration might be more appropriate but this is generally unsatisfactory.

Treatment and drugs did not apparently interfere with the tests but in ten patients there was a reduction in the protein concentrations after chemotherapy and in one patient the proteins became normal after X-irradiation of his superior vena cava obstruction.

The non-specific interference of the cancer markers by other illnesses is important, although in all but one of our patients (who subsequently developed nephrotic syndrome) it was not a problem. Furthermore, this occurs with any marker to some degree. For instance, CEA concentrations above 10 g/l may indicate carcinoma of the bowel but values of 10–40 g/l frequently occur from other diseases (liver regeneration, bronchitis, or even cigarette smoking). Concentrations greater than 40 g/l are usually cancer diagnostic. In the case of the proteins we have studied these non-specific influences (inflammation, pneumonia, etc.) may cause elevation similar to those associated with tumours. However, providing these interfering influences can be identified they can be taken into account when assessing the results. In practice one would review the patient and the tests at an early opportunity after the infection has subsided.

A useful marker should indicate disease at a time when it is still treatable. This has not been assessed in these patients and to do so would require a very large study. CEA has been recognized as a useful marker for carcinoma of the bowel for 10 years but application of its measurement still plays little part in relieving suffering or prolonging life. With the advent of powerful drugs that can influence solid tumour growth these proteins may have a useful place in treatment.

17.3 SERUM PROTEIN CHANGES IN PATIENTS WITH BREAST TUMOURS

Many attempts have been made to find a serum or urinary substance that might be useful for monitoring patients with breast tumours[8,9] and it is probably true to say that none has lasted the test of time and careful scientific scrutiny. It seems as though breast tumours only rarely produce specific substances and cause less changes in the serum proteins than lung tumours.

17.3.1   Introduction, materials and methods

Three serum proteins, haptoglobin—measured by rocket immunoelectro-phoresis[6], pregnancy-associated α_2-glycoprotein (PAG)—measured by rocket immunoelectrophoresis[6], and carcinoembryonic antigen (CEA)—measured by radioimmunoassay[1], have been partially evaluated in patients with breast cancer. The patients studied were those attending a chemotherapy clinic at the Queen Elizabeth Medical Centre. Each patient was examined clinically and radiologically at the time of attendance and each was categorized into one of the usual four clinical stages. Blood samples were collected at each attendance; prior to operation for stage 1 and 2 disease and post-operatively at 4–6 weeks. Control subjects were normal women of comparable age. All samples were stored as serum at −20 °C until analysis.

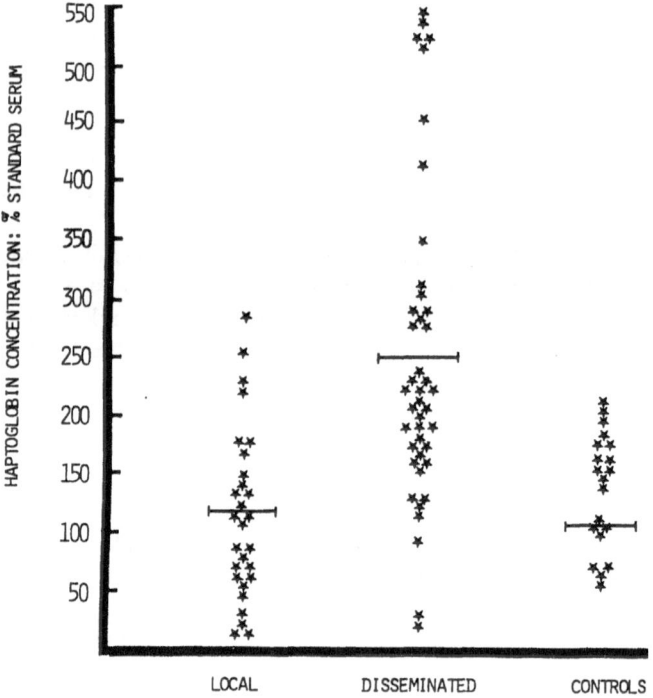

Figure 17.6   Relationship between serum haptoglobin concentrations and breast tumour staging. The bars are the median values

17.3.2 Results

17.3.2.1 Haptoglobin

Haptoglobin concentrations and breast tumour staging are shown in Figure 17.6. There was no significant difference between the protein concentrations in the control group and the patients with stage 1 and 2 tumours but most patients with disseminated disease (stages 3 and 4) had much higher protein concentrations ($p < 0.0005$).

Comparison of the pre-operative and post-operative haptoglobin levels for 15 patients with stage 1 and 2 disease showed no significant change ($p > 0.1$) when using the Wilcoxon paired rank test. However, at 4–6 weeks, some acute phase response could still be influencing the haptoglobin concentrations post-operatively.

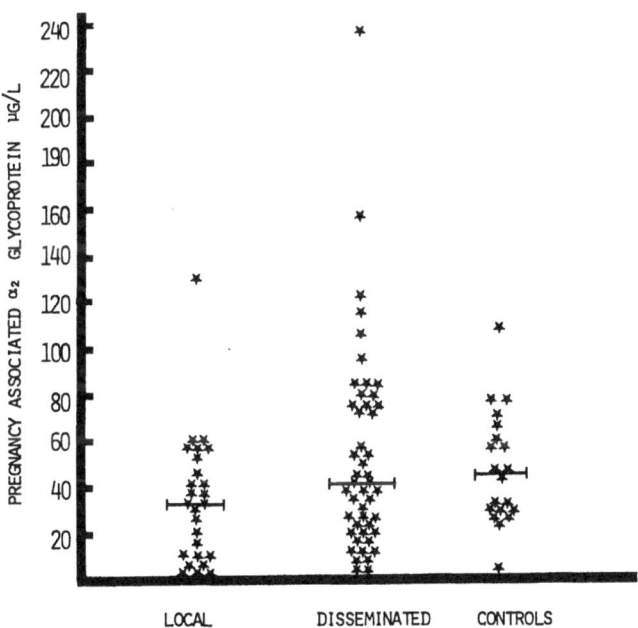

Figure 17.7 Relationship between serum pregnancy-associated α_2-glycoprotein concentrations and breast tumour staging. The bars are the median values

17.3.2.2   *Pregnancy-associated α_2-glycoprotein (PAG)*

The PAG concentrations and breast tumour staging are shown in Figure 17.7. There were no significant differences between the control group of normal women and the patients with localized breast cancer or disseminated breast cancer. However, a few patients did have very high values of PAG but it is doubtful if a group of patients could be usefully monitored by measuring this protein[10].

17.3.2.3   *Carcinoembryonic antigen (CEA)*

Serum CEA concentrations were significantly elevated in patients with stage 1 and 2 cancer ($n=43$, $p= <0.001$) and stage 4 disease ($n=57$, $p<0.001$) when compared with a reference population of 269 healthy subjects (Figure 17.8). Patients with stage 4 disease had significantly higher CEA concentrations

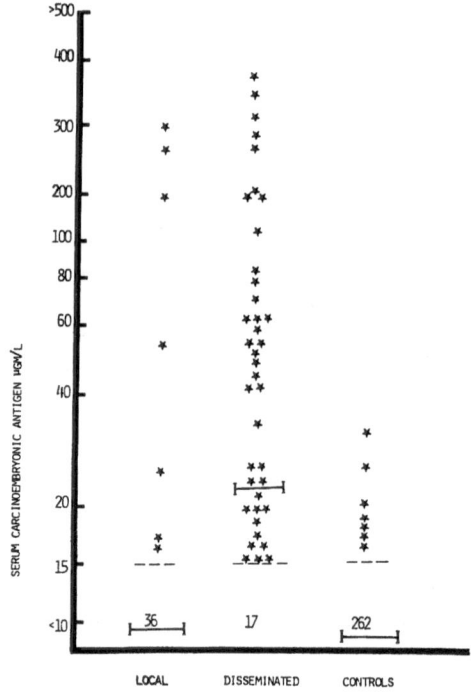

Figure 17.8   Relationship between serum carcinoembryonic antigen concentrations and breast tumour staging. The bars are the median values

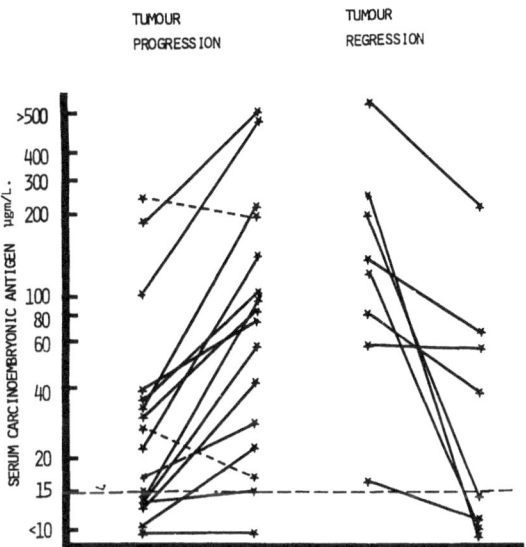

Figure 17.9 Alteration in serum carcinoembryonic antigen concentrations with clinical tumour progression and regression

than the group with stage 1 and 2 disease ($p < 0.001$). CEA concentrations were significantly reduced following excision of primary tumours ($p < 0.05$) and concentrations increased in 15 of the 18 subjects who developed metastases on follow-up ($p < 0.01$) (Figure 17.9). CEA concentrations therefore increase in relation to tumour burden and reflect the progress of metastases.

17.4 CONCLUSION

The results show that significant changes occur in the serum in some patients who have breast and lung tumours but usually the changes tend to be dismissed as 'non-specific'.

This is not synonymous with 'useless' and until the advent of more specific markers these acute phase proteins remain the most sensitive indication of the progress of some tumours. Each protein has a slightly different role. CEA, a specific tumour product when elevated, is probably the most reliable indication of disease. Orosomucoid is less reliable because elevations occur non-specifically; however, it is easier to measure and is abnormal in a greater proportion of patients. Haptoglobin seems to offer no advantage over oroso-mucoid and suffers from the disadvantage that the different phenotypes are qualitatively different when measured immunologically. C-reactive protein is probably no more sensitive than orosomucoid and the advantage that it increases many-fold above normal levels must be weighed against the lack of response that occurs in some patients. It is not as good as orosomucoid in relation to lung tumour size.

Other patients that have been studied include those with large bowel tumours and stomach tumours[11]. The results are less striking than with lung tumours but more marked than in the breast tumour group and the protein concentrations remain high for many months after surgery probably as a result of minor wound sepsis.

In many ways the most curious aspect of these studies is that substances useful for monitoring these patients with cancer have no well-ascribed function.

Acknowledgements

I would like to thank D. Burnett (Department of Immunology, University of Birmingham, Birmingham B15), C. E. Newman and C. H. J. Ford (Surgical Immunology Unit, Department of Surgery, Queen Elizabeth Medical Centre, Birmingham B15 2TH) and D. Cove (Department of Medicine, Dudley Road Hospital, Birmingham B18) for supplying the clinical information and much of the experimental data which have made this article possible. I am also indebted to the many other members of the Departments of Medicine, Surgery and Immunology who have offered helpful advice to the many surgeons and physicians in Birmingham whose patients were studied.

References

1. Booth, S. N., Jamieson, G. C., King, J. P. G., Leonard, J., Oates, G. D. and Dykes, P. W. (1974). Carcinoembryonic antigen in the management of colorectal carcinoma. *Br. Med. J.*, **4**, 183
2. Abelev, G. I., Assecritova, I. U., Kraevsky, N. A., Perova, S. D. and Perevod-chikove, N. I. (1967). Embryonal serum α-globulin in cancer patients: diagnostic value. *Int. J. Cancer*, **2**, 551
3. Bradwell, A. R., Burnett, D., Ford, C. H. J. and Newman, C. E. (1977). Serial measurements of plasma proteins for monitoring patients with carcinoma of the lung. *Clin. Sci. Mol. Med.*, **51**, 21
4. Neville, A. M. and Cooper, E. H. (1976). Biochemical monitoring of cancer. *Ann. Clin. Biochem.*, **13**, 283

5. Newman, C. E., Ford, C. H. J., Davies, D. A. L. and O'Neill,. G.. J. (1977). Antibody–drug sypergism: an assessment of specific passive immunotherapy in bronchial carcinoma. *Lancet,* **ii,** 163
6. Laurell, C–B. (1972). Electroimmunoassay. *Scand. J. Clin. Lab. Invest.,* **129,** Suppl. 124, 21
7. Soorae, A. S. and Abbey-Smith, R. (1976). Tumour size as a prognostic factor after resection of the lung. *Thorax,* **32,** 19
8. Coombes, R. C., Powles, T. J., Gazet, J. C., Ford, H. T., Sloane, J. P., Laurence, D. J. R. and Neville, A. M. (1977). Biochemical markers in human breast cancer. *Lancet,* **i,** 132
9. Cove, D. H., Woods, K. L., Howell, A., Smith, S. C. H., Burnett, D., Bradwell, A. R., Leonard, J. and Heath, D. A. (1977). The evaluation of seven potential tumour markers in human breast cancer. In *Biological and immunological Aspects of Tumour Markers.* (In press)
10. Burnett, D., Booth, S. N., Cove, D. H., Howell, A., Sturdee, D. and Bradwell, A. R. (1977). Pregnancy-associated α_2-glycoprotein. *Lancet,* **i,** 257
11. Milford Ward, A., Cooper, E. H., Turner, R., Anderson, J. A. and Neville, A. M. (1977). Acute phase reactant protein profiles: an aid to monitoring large bowel cancer by CEA and serum enzymes. *Br. J. Cancer,* **35,** 170

SECTION THREE

Immunochemistry of Other Body Fluids

Chairman: Dr J. T. Whicher

18

Urinary proteins
J. Hardwicke

18.1 INTRODUCTION   219

18.2 NORMAL PROTEIN HANDLING   220

18.3 PATHOPHYSIOLOGY   221

18.4 CLINICAL ASPECTS   221
    18.4.1   *Tubular proteinuria*   221
    18.4.2   *Overflow proteinuria*   222
    18.4.3   *Glomerular proteinuria*   224
    18.4.4   *Nephrogenic proteinuria*   224

18.5 CONCLUSION   226

18.1 INTRODUCTION

From the previous chapters in this book it will have become apparent that the strength of immunochemical methods, in the analysis of the complex mixture of macromolecules in biological fluids, lies in the specificity which is available in these, but few other, methods. There is however an inherent disadvantage in this very specificity in that the field of view is inevitably narrow. While immunochemical techniques are very valuable for answering a specific question, such as: 'What are the relative urine:plasma ratios for IgG and transferrin in an individual patient?', they do not give an overall picture of other proteins, also of clinical importance, present in the fluid.

In this chapter I will review the pathophysiology of proteinuria, the most important single clinical sign of renal disease. In elucidating this pathophysiology, immunochemical techniques were of major importance[1], and showed that both quantity and quality of proteinuria vary widely in association with different diseases. They also contributed to the realization that a major factor determining protein excretion in both normal and diseased kidneys is molecular size. With the development, in the early 1970s, of the technique of electrophoresis in polyacrylamide gels containing sodium dodecyl sulphate (SDSPAE)[2], this method, which analyses protein mixtures on the basis of molecular size, is likely to become the major screening technique. Immunochemical analyses will however remain as an important confirmatory method.

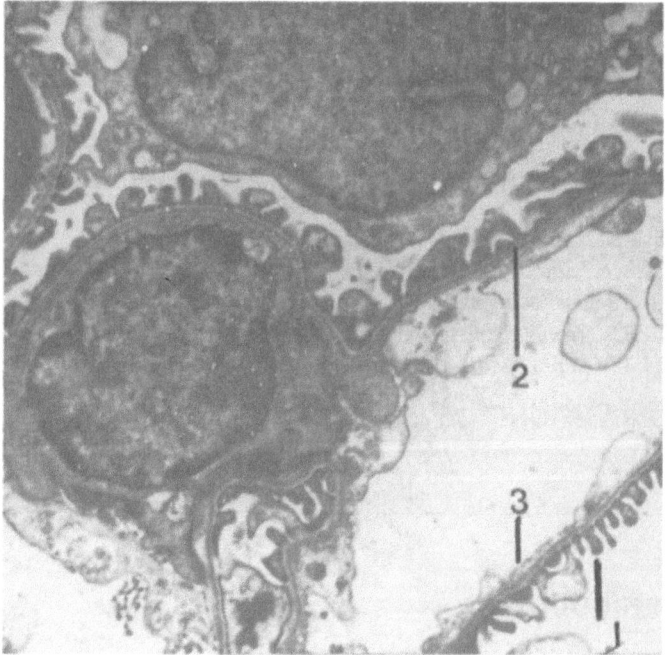

Figure 18.1 Electron micrograph of a normal glomerulus. 1, Epithelial cell with foot processes extending into Bowman's space; 2, Basement membrane; 3, Endothelial cell lining the glomerular capillary

18.2 NORMAL PROTEIN HANDLING

Formation of urine is by a process of plasma ultrafiltration at the glomerulus, and reabsorption by the tubules. Glomerular capillary structure differs from that of peripheral capillaries in three respects (Figure 18.1):

(i) The endothelial cell layer is fenestrated allowing plasma protein direct contact with the basement membrane.

(ii) The basement membrane is thicker, and shows three well defined areas: a central lamina densa, and laminae rarae internal and external to this.

(iii) There are highly specialized epithelial cells, forming a continuous coat over the basement membrane. These have complex interdigitating foot processes with a well marked surface glycocalyx.

Morphological studies, using macromolecules of defined size and rendered electron dense[3], suggest that high molecular weight molecules, such as ferritin, are held up in the lamina densa, while smaller molecules such as albumin are restricted by the slit pores of the epithelial cells. Morphological damage to these, such as occurs in some experimental and human disorders[4], is associated with a heavy proteinuria in which serum albumin preponderates. Other factors that may be of importance are maintenance of blood flow[5] and the isoelectric properties of the macromolecules[6].

Functional studies are based both on direct tubular puncture[7] and also, indirectly, on urine excretion of macromolecules following intravenous infusion[8]. Such studies have shown that the normal transglomerular clearance of albumin is less than 0.02% of the filtration rate, representing a total passage of under 2 g/day. For molecules only slightly smaller than albumin, the clearances increase rapidly with diminishing molecular size.

Reabsorption of protein by the normal tubule undoubtedly occurs, since less than 100 mg/day are passed to the urine. Also, in conditions of proteinuria, protein droplets are found in the proximal tubules. The capacity for such reabsorption is not known, except in relation to the light chains of IgG, where the equivalent of some 50 g/day may be catabolized by the tubules[9].

18.3 PATHOPHYSIOLOGY

From the considerations above it is possible to predict four mechanisms by which protein can be lost into the urine—all of these have now been described:

(i) *Tubular proteinuria*—damage to the tubule leading to the loss of proteins present in the normal filtrate.

(ii) *Overflow proteinuria*—loss of protein filtered by the normal glomerulus in amounts sufficient to saturate normal tubular reabsorption. Such protein, by definition, must be more readily filtered, and therefore smaller, than albumin.

(iii) *Glomerular proteinuria*—abnormal permeability of glomerular capillaries, with leakage of normal plasma proteins.

(iv) *Nephrogenic proteinuria*—the above three arise by a process of filtration, but in addition protein might be added to the filtrate in its passage down the nephron. This can be termed nephrogenic proteinuria.

In any individual patient these types are not mutually exclusive, and such mixed proteinurias then give some indication of the nature of the functional lesion in the nephron.

18.4   CLINICAL ASPECTS

18.4.1   Tubular proteinuria

Figure 18.2 shows an SDSPAE separation of serum and urine from a patient with tubular proteinuria. Four separate protein bands are seen migrating faster than albumin, and are therefore smaller. The estimation of individual proteins, including lysozyme[10] and β_2-microglobulin[11], has been used in the past as an indicator of tubular proteinuria. These small proteins are reabsorbed independently of albumin and the larger plasma proteins, since they are often not found in patients with heavy glomerular proteinuria, a condition in which tubular reabsorption capacity for protein must be saturated (Figure 18.4). The patient illustrated in Figure 18.2 had pyelonephritis, a condition often associated in our experience with tubular proteinuria—the presence of traces of IgG in the urine suggest that there is also a glomerular element.

18.4.2   Overflow proteinuria

The classical example of this type of proteinuria is the excretion of monoclonal light chains in Bence Jones proteinuria. Figure 18.3 illustrates one such case, where the light-chain excretion is as a monomer of about 34 000 daltons.

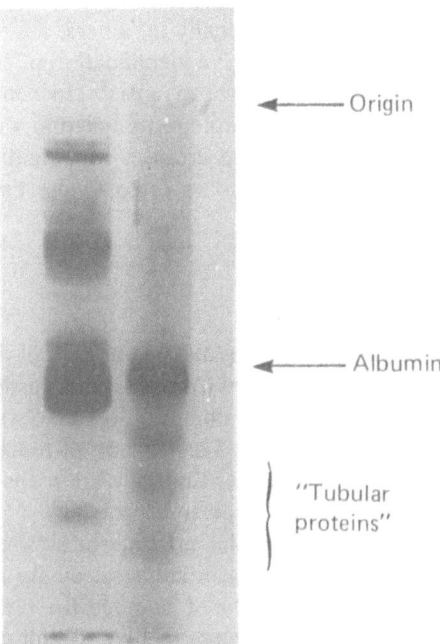

Figure 18.2   SDSPAE of serum and urine from a case of pyelonephritis with tubular proteinuria

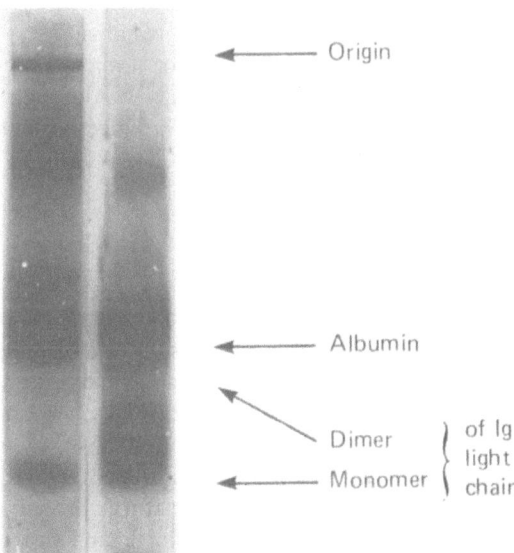

Figure 18.3   SDSPAE of serum and urine showing overflow proteinuria in a Bence Jones myeloma

More commonly dimers, and occasionally tetramers, are excreted[12]. Immuno-electrophoresis is necessary for positive identification of the monoclonal light chain, and this may be important in prognosis[13]. In some cases of myeloid leukaemia, lysozyme is lost in the urine in association with very high serum levels, and several groups of workers are now investigating the loss into the urine of polypeptides related to tumours or to severe tissue damage[14].

18.4.3 Glomerular proteinuria

Any disease associated with glomerular damage will lead to glomerular proteinuria, though the quantity varies from less than 1 g/day to over 30 g/day. The major urinary protein is usually albumin (Figure 18.4) and the proportion of globulins varies from case to case. The absence of tubular proteins, smaller than albumin, is striking, and indicates that they are reabsorbed by a different mechanism from that of the major plasma proteins.

Studies on the quality of glomerular proteinuria have concentrated on the relative protein clearances[15]. In all cases some selectivity by molecular size is retained, but with increasing severity of damage the clearance of IgG and larger molecules, such as $\alpha_2 M$, increases relative to that of albumin or trans-ferrin. These particular plasma proteins show clearances closely related to molecular size[15], but other plasma proteins do not always behave as expected from their estimated molecular size[16]. The clearance of IgG relative to trans-ferrin has proved a useful predictor of steroid responsiveness[15] (Table 18.1). More recently we have described a tendency for urinary albumin to dimerize in patients who are responding to steroid therapy[17]. Although the mechanism for this is not yet understood, it promises to be an even better predictor of steroid responsiveness than the IgG clearance (Table 18.2).

18.4.4 Nephrogenic proteinuria

Protein can be added to the ultrafiltrate either by normal processes of secretion, or by loss from the structural elements of the nephron. In the first category is the Tamm-Horsfall glycoprotein[18], a normal urinary constituent of unknown function, and a major constituent of casts[19]. Also secretory IgA has been reported in association with renal tract infection, though this has yet to prove clinically useful[20]. There have been a number of reports of the excretion of both tubular and glomerular structural proteins in health and disease[21,22], but the estimation of these is difficult, and has yet to prove of value in following disease activity.

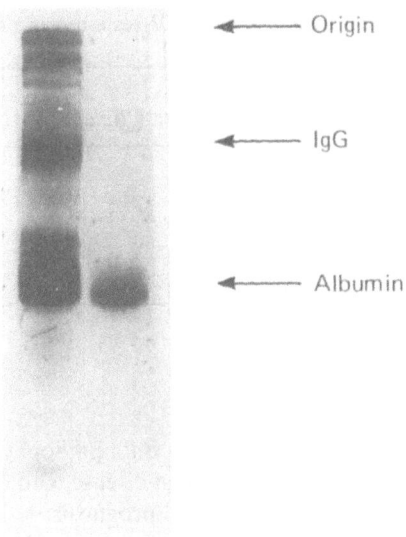

Figure 18.4   SDSPAE of serum and urine showing a glomerular proteinuria

**TABLE 18.1   Correlation of IgG/transferrin clearance
with steroid response**

IgG (% transferrin) clearance	% responding
0–10	80
11–15	58
16–20	35
21–30	25
over 31	less than 5

TABLE 18.2   Albumin polymer and steroid response in children

Polymer	Number	Responders	Relapsing	Dependent	Unresponsive
Positive	15	15	0	0	0
Negative	13	1	1	3	8

18.5   CONCLUSION

The identification of types of proteinuria on a pathophysiological basis makes it possible to assess the sites of damage in disease, and on occasions to predict response to therapy and make ultimate prognosis.

While, in most cases, the analysis of the proteinuria concurs with our knowledge of pathophysiological mechanisms, there are a number of unresolved anomalies. The further study of such anomalies may well add to our knowledge both of plasma proteins and of the pathology of renal disease. In such studies there is no doubt that immunochemistry will play an important role[23].

References

1. Hardwicke, J. (1970). Proteinuria. In *Scientific Basis of Medicine Annual Reviews*. p. 211. (The Athlone Press, University of London)
2. Waldmann, T. A., Strober, W. and Mogieluicki, R. P. (1972). Renal handling of low molecular weight proteins. *J. Clin. Invest.*, **51**, 2162
3. Farquhar, M. G. (1975). The primary glomerular filtration barrier. Basement membrane or epithelial slits. *Kidney Int.*, **8**, 197
4. Powell, H. R. (1976). Relationship between proteinuria and epithelial cell changes in minimal lesion glomerulopathy. *Nephron*, **16**, 319
5. Ryan, G. B. and Karnovsky, M. J. (1976). Distribution of endogenous albumin in the rat glomerulus: role of haemodynamic factors in glomerular barrier function. *Kidney Int.*, **9**, 36
6. Rennke, H. and Venkatachalam, M. A. (1977). Glomerular permeability: *in vivo* tracer studies with polyanionic and polycationic ferritins. *Kidney Int.*, **11**, 44
7. Landwehr, D. M., Carvalho, J. S. and Oken, D. E. (1977). Micropuncture studies of the filtration and absorption of albumin by nephrotic rats. *Kidney Int.*, **11**, 9
8. Hulme, B. and Hardwicke, J. (1968). Human glomerular permeability to macromolecules in health and disease. *Clin. Sci.*, **34**, 515

9. Waldmann, T. and Strober, W. (1973). Renal regulation of serum protein metabolism. In: H. Peeters (ed.). *Protides of Biological Fluids*. Vol. 21, p. 419. (Oxford: Pergamon Press)

10. Harrison, J. F. and Blainey, J. D. (1967). Low molecular weight proteinuria in chronic renal disease. *Clin. Sci.*, **33**, 381

11. Berggard, I. and Bearn, A. G. (1968). Isolation and properties of a low molecular weight β_2 globulin in biological fluids. *J. Biol. Chem.*, **243**, 4095

12. Harrison, J. F., Blainey, J. D., Hardwicke, J., Rowe, D. S. and Soothill, J. F. (1966). Proteinuria in multiple myeloma. *Clin. Sci.*, **31**, 95

13. McLaughlin, H. and Hobbs, J. R. (1972). Clinical significance of Bence-Jones proteinuria. In Peeters, H. (ed.). *Protides of Biological Fluids*, Vol. 20, p. 251. (Oxford: Pergamon Press)

14. Antoine, B. and Neveu, T. (1970). Tissue-like macromolecules in pathological urine (histuria). In Manuel, Y., Revillard, J. P. and Betuel, J. (eds.). *Proteins in Normal and Pathological Urine*, p. 244. (New York: S. Karger)

15. Hardwicke, J., Cameron, J. S., Harrison, J. R., Hulme, B. and Soothill, J. F. (1970). Proteinuria in kidney disease. In Manuel, Y., Revillard, J. P. and Betuel, H. (eds.). *Proteins in Normal and Pathological Urine*, p. 111. (New York: S. Karger)

16. Bienenstock, J. and Poortmans, J. (1970). Renal clearances of fifteen plasma proteins in diseases. *J. Lab. Clin. Med.*, **75**, 297

17. Boesken, W. H., Schindera, F., Billingham, M., Hardwicke, J., White, R. H. R. and Williams, A. (1977). Polymeric albumin in the urine of patients with nephrotic syndrome. *Clin, Nephrol.*, **8**, 395

18. Maxfield, M. (1961). Molecular forms of urinary mucoprotein present under physiological conditions. *Biochem. Biophys. Acta*, **49**, 548

19. McQueen, E. G. (1962). The nature of urinary casts. *J. Clin. Pathol.*, **15**, 367

20. Tomasi, T. B. Jr. and Bienenstock, J. (1968). Secretory immunoglobulins. *Adv. Immunol.*, **9**, 21

21. Mondorf, A. W., Carpenter, C. B., Scherberich, J. E. and Merril, J. P. (1973). Specific tubular histuria following transplantation. In Peeters, H. (ed.). *Protides of Biological Fluids*, Vol. 21, p. 493. (Oxford: Pergamon Press)

22. Batsford, S. R. and Hardwicke, J. (1975). The spectrum of urinary basement membrane antigen excretion in normal and pathological rabbit urine. *Clin. Nephrol.*, **3**, 60

23. Hardwicke, J. (1975). Laboratory aspects of proteinuria. *Clin. Nephrol.*, **3**, 37

19

Immunochemistry of CSF proteins
E. J. Thompson

19.1	INTRODUCTION	229
19.2	PHYSIOLOGY	230
	19.2.1 Production, circulation and reabsorption of CSF	230
	19.2.2 CSF protein metabolism	230
19.3	CSF PROTEINS IN DISEASE	231
19.4	ROUTINE LABORATORY INVESTIGATION OF CSF	233
19.5	EXAMINATION OF THE GAMMAGLOBULINS	233
	19.5.1 Estimation of IgG	233
	19.5.2 Visualization of the gammaglobulins	234
19.6	CONCLUSION	236

19.1 INTRODUCTION

Qualitative and quantitative examination of the proteins in cerebrospinal fluid (CSF) may be very helpful in the diagnosis of certain neurological diseases such as disseminated sclerosis.

19.2 PHYSIOLOGY

The physiology of CSF protein metabolism is in many ways unique and an understanding is essential to interpretation of changes occurring in disease.

19.2.1 Production, circulation and reabsorption of CSF

The CSF is produced primarily in the choroid plexus of each of the lateral ventricles and the third and fourth ventricles and is absorbed primarily in a quite distant site, the arachnoid villi, which protrudes into the superior sagittal sinus. Additional reabsorption also occurs into the capillary circulation of the membranes surrounding the CSF and into tissue cells.

During its circuitous course, the CSF is propelled in part by the action of the cilia from the ependymal cells and also in part by the pulsation of the brain during each heart beat. The CSF passes from the lateral ventricles, through into the third ventricle, down the aqueduct into the fourth ventricle and up over the cortex as well as down surrounding the spinal cord. The spinal cord constitutes, in effect, a cul-de-sac, and therefore the flow of CSF is confronted by a dead-end.

19.2.2 CSF protein metabolism

The production of CSF involves primarily a filtration effect in which approximately one molecule in 200 is allowed passage through the choroid plexus, and passage of each particular molecule is mainly based on its size. There is a striking difference in size between IgG and albumin, the immunoglobulin molecule being more than twice as large as albumin. Immunoglobulin constitutes 3–5% of total CSF protein[1] but 15–19% of total serum protein. This reflects the sieving action of the choroid plexus barrier. One might expect a linear relationship between the relative abundance of particular proteins in the CSF (compared with that in the serum) and the average molecular size. In fact, this linear relationship between relative abundance and molecular size is only seen in the case of high levels of CSF total protein. In the lower (normal) levels of total protein one sees a slight deviation from linearity in the case of not only IgG but also IgA, in which these proteins are relatively excluded by the choroid plexes[2]. The normal barrier for the production of CSF is dramatically altered in the first few months of life as well as in patients who are over 65, although the alteration is less striking in the older age group.

There is typically a 300% difference between the level of total protein found in the lumbar sac and that found within the ventricles. Furthermore, there is a striking difference in the composition of the individual proteins which make up the total protein level. Within the ventricles the prominent proteins are low molecular weight pre-albumin and albumin. By contrast, the lumbar fluid is conspicuous by the prominence of high molecular weight proteins. This reflects the progressive equilibration of the poorly circulating spinal fluid with plasma through the capillaries of the meninges. This is exaggerated in spinal blocks where there is no circulation of CSF below the lesion, and as time passes such CSF comes progressively to resemble plasma in both the level of total protein and the pattern of proteins present.

19.3   CSF PROTEINS IN DISEASE

The concentrations of proteins in the plasma clearly influence the amount present in the CSF as the filtration of proteins by the choroid plexus is dependent on both size and concentration. It is thus important when considering the concentrations of proteins such as IgG or albumin in CSF to take account of the serum levels. Various quotients have been derived to relate CSF levels to serum levels and thus eliminate the effect of varying serum concentrations on levels in the CSF[3]. The changes seen in CSF proteins in disease may be divided into a number of groups:

(a) Increased passage of plasma proteins into the CSF:
(i) Increased capillary permeability. This occurs in acute inflammatory conditions such as bacterial and viral meningitis and lupus erythematosus. It also occurs in some chronic inflammatory conditions, intracranial malignancies and cerebrovascular disease.
(ii) Mechanical obstruction. In these conditions progressive equilibration of static CSF with plasma occurs. The same picture is seen in the Guillain-Barré syndrome.

(b) Patterns reflecting plasma protein changes. The changes of paraproteinaemia, Bence Jones proteinaemia, cirrhosis and nephrotic syndrome are all reflected in the CSF.

(c) Local immunoglobulin production in the central nervous system. This may be seen in:
(i) Chronic infectious diseases such as neurosyphilis, tuberculous meningitis, trypanosomiasis and others
(ii) Disseminated sclerosis
(iii) Subacute sclerosing panencephalitis.

It is in the investigation of CSF immunoglobulin production that the influence of increased capillary permeability and serum immunoglobulin levels must be eliminated. This is usually achieved by measuring CSF IgG along with albumin as a measure of capillary permeability and correcting for the serum levels of both proteins. A quotient may thus be derived from the ratio of the CSF/serum IgG to the CSF/serum albumin. This quotient is in fact a clearance ratio and high levels reflect synthesis of IgG within the CSF space.

Disseminated sclerosis is by far the most important disease in this group and will be used as an example of the processes which may occur. Three distinct pathological processes occur in the region of the perivascular cuff:

(a) the transudate of serum IgG which occurs due to local destruction of the barrier, namely, the wall of the vein.

(b) the local occurrence of plasma cells with direct synthesis of IgG in the contiguous environment.

(c) local destruction of immunoglobulins to produce fragments, including free light chains, and also various other fragments of tissue including myelin. The pathological CSF IgG is more cathodic than the IgG from the corresponding serum, and since polyacrylamide has the striking ability to sieve proteins on a basis of their molecular size, it is a reasonable first assumption that this difference is due to an aggregated association of the immunoglobulin with either another immunoglobulin (or fragment) or a specific antigen.

(d) Patterns due to removal of sialic acid from proteins. During the course of CSF circulation there is a normal alteration of a number of glycoproteins (orosomucoid, α_1-antitrypsin, hemopexin and transferrin) due to the removal of sialic acid residues by enzymes present on the periventricular and other surfaces. These changes generally result in a decreased electrophoretic mobility and in the case of transferrin the more cathodal form is known as the tau protein. This is immunologically identical and therefore complicates any simple precipitin reaction based upon antibodies raised to transferrin. Analysis of ventricular fluid also confirms the low amount of tau protein in this region of the brain. This is consistent with the fact that the tau protein has been produced from the serum transferrin, which has only recently been filtered by the choroid plexus. The level of the tau protein can be further increased in those situations which give rise to abnormal stasis in CSF flow, such as is seen in alcoholic degenerative processes. Although the tau protein could be visualized as a protein which is specific to the nervous system in the sense that it is produced by the normal actions of the periventricular and other surfaces on the transferrin, once again its amount is a function of the normal flow rate, and as such can be altered in secondary fashion, depending upon whether or not one has obstructive hydrocephalus or even communicating hydrocephalus.

19.4   ROUTINE LABORATORY INVESTIGATION OF CSF

The tests which are actually performed at our hospital include the following:

(1) Determination of total protein, using a nephelometric technique based upon the precipitation of proteins using polyethylene glycol.

(2) The qualitative assessment of immunoglobulin excess, using the Pandy technique of saturated phenol. This should always be negative if the total protein is less than 0.8 grams per litre.

(3) The Lange colloidal gold curve is also used as a qualitative assessment, looking particularly for the first zone or paretic curve which has predictive value for an elevated slow gamma[4].

(4) Quantitative estimation of CSF and serum IgG, IgA, IgM and albumin using radial immunodiffusion. Agarose electrophoresis of serum is also performed.

(5) Qualitative examination of the immunoglobulins by polyacrylamide gel electrophoresis. No stacking gel or sucrose is used; 100 μg of protein are applied to one gel stained with Coomassie blue and 200 μl of protein to a second gel stained with Naphthol black. This gives one a comparison between the two gels for the gammaglobulins, since Coomassie is known to give twice as much binding to IgG (relative to albumin) as does Naphthol. Elevated amounts of slow gamma can then be confirmed by direct immunofixation with the appropriate antibodies on the surface of the gel.

19.5   EXAMINATION OF THE GAMMAGLOBULINS

19.5.1   Estimation of IgG

IgG is commonly determined by immunoprecipitation in various forms:

(a) Mancini radial immunodiffusion.

(b) Laurell rocket electroimmunodiffusion.

(c) Nephelometric determination of the light scattered by the immuno-precipitates.

Although CSF IgG was first estimated by electrophoresis[5], this required some 70 ml of CSF, and immunoprecipitation methods were introduced in which only 1 ml was required[6]. Since current electrophoretic methods require only 0.5 ml or less, the pendulum has begun to swing the other way. Normally one only requires a few μl to estimate IgG by immunoprecipitation, but again, one is looking at a specified protein rather than seeking a complete profile of all of the CSF proteins. Some of the problems which are associated with the determination of IgG by immunoprecipitation can be enumerated as follows:

(a) The apparent IgG determined by this method may be much higher than the amount of intact immunoglobulin. In a given patient the CSF IgG may be estimated as 45% of the total protein, using immunoprecipitation techniques, whereas in fact on electrophoresis it may be in the range of 25% of total protein, the difference being made up both by fragments of immunoglobulins and by free light chains[7].

(b) Another problem which is commonly seen is the occurrence of double rings, due to the fact that the lower molecular weight fragments diffuse faster and form an outer ring, whereas the intact molecules form an inner ring due to their larger size, and consequently their slower rate of diffusion.

(c) Such methodological problems may contribute to the fact that the discriminating value of the CSF/serum IgG : albumin clearance ratio is by no means perfect for the diagnosis of disseminated sclerosis. In collaboration with Dr Pamela Riches at the Supra-Regional Protein Reference Unit at Queen Mary Hospital, Putney, we have looked at 29 patients in this way and found one false positive and six false negatives. Admittedly, these were patients selected as being in the rather difficult area of intermediate values, but, nonetheless, it underlines the difficulties which are inherent in a method which simply measures two proteins. Better discrimination can be obtained by examination of the CSF gammaglobulin on polyacrylamide gel electrophoresis.

19.5.2 Visualization of the gammaglobulins

Because of the unique sieving nature of polyacrylamide gel electrophoresis, it is more useful for qualitative examination of gammaglobulins than the older, non-sieving media such as paper, cellulose acetate, agar or agarose. Slow (cathodic) gamma has the additional property of increased molecular size on polyacrylamide or starch gel which is not important for the other media. Acrylamide can comfortably cope with 40–50 bands whereas the other media separate only about 6–10 bands.

The gammaglobulin region is conventionally divided into five portions as shown in Figure 19.1, and the oligoclonal pattern is defined as the occurrence of at least three diffuse bands in which the primary band is not in the gamma-1 position, and further that one does not have principal sharp bands of gamma-2 and gamma-4, as seen with haemoglobin–haptoglobin complexes due to a traumatic tap. This is not to be confused with the sharp bands due to haptoglobin oligomers (auto-polymers of the monomer). Using these criteria, more than 90% of patients with multiple sclerosis have a positive oligoclonal pattern on polyacrylamide gel electrophoresis. It has also been found that increasing amounts of slow gamma correlate with the clinical status

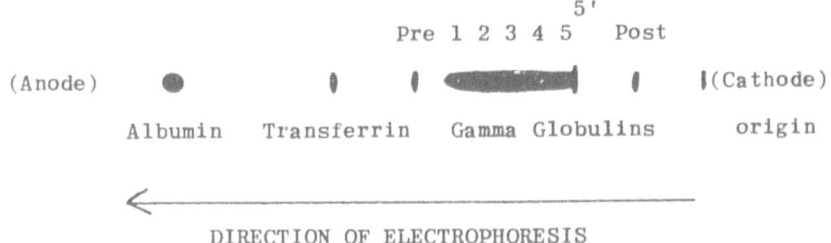

Figure 19.1 Diagrammatic representation of subdivision of gamma region into five areas. Double band in the region five is termed 5

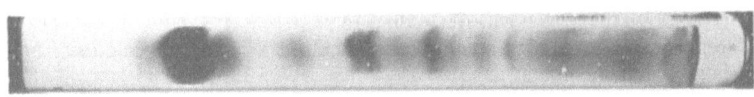

Figure 19.2 Polyacrylamide gel of CSF from patient with multiple sclerosis. Total protein 1.0 g/l; cathode on right; gel length 13 cm

of the patient in that the more certain the clinical diagnosis, the higher the amount of cathodic IgG. If one is attempting to assess the effects of steroids (such as may be given to a patient with multiple sclerosis) upon the levels of IgG within the spinal fluid, one must distinguish the two effects of the steroids:

(1) The decreased transudative leakage of proteins. This is due to the fact that the inflammatory response destroys the normal blood–CSF barrier by which the vessels filter serum proteins, and the anti-inflammatory action of steroids helps to restore the normal barrier.

(2) The immunosuppression of local plasma cells in their synthesis of IgG. This CSF pattern is seen in Figure 19.2, which illustrates both the high molecular weight haptoglobin oligomers, due to transudation (also manifesting itself as an elevation in the total protein), and the diffuse elevation of IgG in the gamma-5 region due to local synthesis. The increased gamma-5 has also been investigated in patients with disseminated sclerosis who have been studied longitudinally. During exacerbation of the disease this particular slow gamma fraction shows a further elevation.

19.6 CONCLUSION

In summary, one can say that CSF/serum IgG:albumin clearance may provide a simple basis and perhaps the minimum investigation for the correct interpretation of spinal fluid levels of immunoglobulins, but that the most satisfactory answers will come from the complete analysis of all of the CSF proteins by the more discriminating technique of polyacrylamide gel electrophoresis.

References

1. Schliep, G., Rapic, N. and Felgenhauer, K. (1974). Quantitation of high molecular proteins in cerebrospinal fluid. *Z. Klin. Chem. Klin. Biochem.*, **12**, 367
2. Felgenhauer, K., Schliep, G. and Rapic, N. (1976). Evaluation of the blood–CSF barrier by protein gradients and the humoral immune response within the central nervous system. *J. Neurol. Sci.*, **30**, 113
3. Thompson, E. J. (1977). Laboratory diagnosis of multiple sclerosis: immunological and biochemical aspects. *Br. Med. Bull.*, **33**, (1), 28
4. Thompson, E. J., Norman, P. M. and MacDermot, J. (1975). The analysis of cerebrospinal fluid. *Br. J. Hosp. Med.*, **14**, 645
5. Kabat, E. A., Moore, D. H. and Landow, H. (1942). An electrophoretic study of the protein components in cerebrospinal fluid and their relationship to the serum proteins. *J. Clin. Invest.*, **21**, 571
6. Kabat, E. A., Glusman, M. and Knaub, V. (1948). Quantitative estimation of the albumin and gammaglobulin in normal and pathologic cerebrospinal fluid by immunochemical methods. *Am. J. Med.*, **IV**, (5), 653
7. Bollengier, F., Delmotte, P. and Lowenthal, A. (1976). Biochemical findings in multiple sclerosis. III. Immunoglobulins of restricted heterogeneity and light chain distribution in cerebrospinal fluid of patients with multiple sclerosis. *J. Neurol.*, **212**, 151

Discussion

This edited version of the discussion which followed the various presentations is included in the Proceedings to bring out some of the more important problems and queries which were raised and discussed at the time. It is not intended to be a complete transcript of the discussion as many of the points raised are covered in detail in the text.

DISCUSSION

SECTION ONE
Methods and Problems in Immunochemistry
Chairmen: Dr A. Milford Ward and Dr A. R. Bradwell

Dr Gillian BLUNDELL (Edinburgh): In immunofixation, can the antiserum solution be re-used or must it be discarded after each fixation?

Dr RICHES: The antiserum solution can be re-used many times. It tends to get contaminated, but it could be filtered through a 0.2 micron millipore filter and cleaned up, one can then dilute more antiserum, and it maintains a reservoir.

Dr H. G. M. FREEMAN (London): Dr Whicher spoke about paraprotein and the problem with antigen excess. Has he run into any problems of non-recognition of antigen excess in polyclonal immunoglobulin measurement?

Dr WHICHER: No. This is not a problem with the polyclonal immuno-globulin increases in the currently available nephelometric systems.

Dr Helen GRIMES (Galway): In the laboratory it is very muddling when commercial firms each maintain that they have standardized their standards against the accepted standard. It would be of considerable help if the commercial firms would agree on a standard.

Dr WHICHER: All commercial manufacturers now state up to three sets of values in their literature; the international units, g/l based on their non-standardization and g/l based on the WHO recommended conversion from international units. Clearly, if weight values are to be used, the most satisfactory will be that derived from international units based on the WHO standard. The WHO standard is unsuitable for nephelometry but other standards which have been calibrated against the WHO are becoming available.

Dr David BURNETT (Birmingham): Not only are there problems in comparing standard sera from different firms, but there is even a problem of differing standards within one particular firm. One company producing both standard plasma and standard serum claims a quoted value for C4 which is 25° higher in the plasma than in the serum. In fact I measured the serum value maybe more than 100% higher than the value in the plasma if another manufacturer's antiserum is used. It is most important to take possible antiserum effects into consideration.

SECTION TWO

Scientific Proteins in Laboratory Diagnosis

Chairmen: Mr D. Browning, Dr R. S. H. Pumphrey, Dr J. Kohn, Professor J. Hardwicke, Dr A. C. Munro

Mr KENNY: Would Dr Kohn comment further on the finding of transient paraprotein in very young infants. Has he found non-transient paraproteins in children of that age, or indeed in children of any age?

Dr KOHN: Transient paraproteins are a phenomenon that can only be observed for a limited time. Mr Kenny is really asking whether malevolent paraproteins can be seen in a child. They have been described in children with immune deficiencies, but fortunately they are very rare.

There is a parallel. Horses that are immunized with pneumococcal vaccines – particularly in the old days – do produce transient paraproteinaemia. Occasionally on vaccination, particularly hyperimmunization, in humans these transient paraproteins have been seen to appear. There are some viral conditions producing monoclonal proteinaemias. For example, the Aleution mink disease is of viral origin. Some years ago Mitchell suggested that he could isolate a filterable virus from the marrow of a myeloma patient which could induce myeloma in mice. This has never been confirmed.

Dr MUNRO: Presumably anaphylactic transfusion reactions involving IgA are mediated by IgE class antibodies. How relevant are Mr Holt's test systems in measuring IgG and IgM class antibodies?

Mr HOLT: I can only quote the literature saying that in all cases the anti-IgA antibody that has caused anaphylactic transfusion reactions has been high titre and easily demonstrable as an IgG class of antibody in the serum.

Dr MUNRO: I have read that – but I think it is surprising.

Mr HOLT: As yet, in our investigations, we have not found a case of a transfusion reaction of this type being caused by anti-IgA, but we are waiting for that eventuality. We are sure it will occur. It certainly has occurred in many countries, and probably in the UK too, but we have been unable to detect it.

Dr Anne MOFFATT (Guildford): Has Professor Jacobs looked at ferritin levels in pregnancy?

Professor JACOBS: Yes. There are some very interesting data. If women are followed-up throughout pregnancy, say from 16 weeks to term, then they start off with a normal serum ferritin and it drops down to iron-deficient levels. This is almost universal in pregnancy. It gets down to iron-deficient levels at about 30 weeks. If they are supplemented with iron, then the levels come down and level out, which is more or less what one would expect to happen.

Mr R. A. CROCKSON (Birmingham): Professor Jacobs has said that serum ferritin behaves as acute phase reactant protein. It is interesting that haptoglobin, another acute phase reactant protein, falls in the way that he suggests that serum ferritin falls during pregnancy.

Could there be any connection in this sort of behaviour?

Professor JACOBS: I do not know. The fall in serum ferritin seems to be related to the amount of iron that is put into the woman. The fall is related to no-iron therapy. If iron therapy is given than the fall is very rapidly reversed.

Professor HARDWICKE: Has Dr Smith tried at all with the difference effect of albumin polymers? All the commercial preparations of freeze-dried albumin contain up to 15–20% of dimer and I have always been worried by whether the dimer in them will give a different value as a standard value compared with what is essentially monomeric in serum.

Dr SMITH: The group in America who made the recommendations on albumin standardization looked at this and they found that it did not have a great effect on the albumin as measured. It could be a problem in some sera where there are very high concentrations.

Dr KOHN: I believe that Dr Smith was involved for quite some time in the non-method factors influencing the estimation of proteins, and of albumin in particular. This is something that can in fact introduce a much bigger error than any of the others.

Dr SMITH: Yes, there are many non-method variables. Posture is probably the major contributory factor in the total non-method variation and may give rise to up to 10–15% variation in the serum albumin.

Dr BURNETT: Dr Whicher mentioned the problem of *in vitro* activation of complement after a blood sample has been collected. Considering the lengthy period of time that quite often elapses between collecting a sample and assaying it, this may be quite a considerable problem, particularly with serum samples where one is waiting for the serum to clot, and the clotting mechanism may itself affect the complement system.

Is there a case here for measuring complement factors in plasma, and would there be any advantage in perhaps having protease inhibitors to try and block the continued cascade after collection?

Dr WHICHER: The answer is 'yes' to both. Ideally one would like to have EDTA plasma, and we try to get this. One reason is the obvious reason that Dr Burnett has mentioned. The other reason is that this allows one also to look at fragments of C3 if one wishes to do so, in an EDTA sample, something which one could never do in a serum sample.

As regards adding protease inhibitors, several people have done it. We did it for a period. It does not make much difference if EDTA plasma is used. It would probably make some slight difference if one intends to store it for a long time. But I would certainly commend to people that they use EDTA plasma if they can. particularly if they use Mancini.

Mr David G. GARRICK (Manchester): Could I take up Dr Whicher on the problem of *in vitro* activation of the complement. It may be rather a naive viewpoint, but surely when one samples some blood and takes an aliquot of serum, there is a limited quantity of C3 and there will not be any manufacture of C3. Hopefully there will not be complete disintegration of it. I believe that the plates that we use in our laboratory are impregnated with anti-C3c, therefore they are only setting out to detect the breakdown products, therefore if one waits for them all to break down, one can detect the breakdown products. Is that rather a naive point?

Dr WHICHER: The C antigen is one of the antigens on the native molecule, together with about four or five others. When it breaks down to get the lower molecular weight fragment of C3c, which is basically still a dimer, but shorter, one is still dealing with a C antigen. So the C antigen is in fact on the native molecule, and on the breakdown product. This has considerably greater antibody consumption for some reason – presumably because this is probably reacting with other things which the so-called C3 antiserum may contain, but this is an antiserum problem. But it also has a much greater mobility in the gel. The overestimation is largely a mobility phenomenon, and it is difficult to explain because different things happen in rockets. All that I can do is to provide empirical evidence. Quite a lot of study has been done. If a sample of serum is left in an incubator at 37 °C overnight, and measured the next day – try it – the published figures suggest about somewhere between 50 and 100% overestimation of C3, using an antibody directed against C3c.

Mr CROCKSON: Dr Whicher is suggesting using EDTA plasma. Would he also advocate using EDTA buffer in the rocket plates, or in the two-dimensional plates? I understand that one gets activation even during electrophoresis.

Dr WHICHER: It is absolutely vital. It is certainly vital for doing two-dimensionals. The degree of activation is dependent upon the batch or the make of agarose used; the agarose is a polysaccharide. and is quite good at activating the alternative pathway. We do use EDTA in the gel and buffer for all electrophoretic techniques involving complement components.

Mr CROCKSON: Which commercial manufacturers put EDTA into their plates?

Dr WHICHER: As far as Mancini is concerned, I do not know. But if an EDTA plasma is used, almost certainly there will be enough EDTA present in the diffusing ring to stop the problem arising on Mancini. It is not adequate on a two-dimensional because there is a much bigger spread.

Dr M. K. C. CHAN (Liverpool): When a high maternal AFP level has been obtained, would Dr Brock differentiate the fetus affected by neural tube defect from that of the low birthweight by the amniotic AFP?

Dr BROCK: Essentially yes. The low birthweight has no abnormality of amniotic fluid AFP.

Dr CHAN: Have there been problems with pregnancies, with amniocentesis, of doing the AFP in amniotic fluid? Presumably the pregnancy with the low birthweight fetus may well be abnormal, or are there no differences found at all?

Dr BROCK: In the low birthweight group which I showed, we were excluding some obvious reasons for low birthweight such as twin pregnancy, or a neural tube defect, or a spontaneous abortion. We were in fact talking about low birthweights which were otherwise normal.

Dr H. G. M. FREEMAN (London): Consider for a moment alpha$_1$ antitrypsin as an acute phase protein. Do the different types of alpha$_1$ antitrypsin respond differently in this situation?

Dr MILFORD WARD: The present evidence is that all the phenotypes respond in a very similar fashion, either to acute tissue injury, or to that other problem with antitrypsin, oestrogen. The percentage elevation of an M type, for example, to oestrogen, is something like 150–200% increase. So the patient or individual receiving oestrogen will have a normal level of around 3 g/l rather than 2.

Take an MZ with a normal level of 1 g/l, put her on oestrogen and the level will rise to 1.5–2 g/l, or about the same proportionate increase.

SECTION THREE

Immunochemistry of Other Body Fluids

Chairman: Dr J. T. Whicher

Dr WHICHER: Professor Hardwicke showed evidence from selectivity studies in children about responsiveness to steroids. What value does he think selectivity studies have in adults with nephrotic syndrome or proteinuria?

Professor HARDWICKE: I think they have roughly the same values as they have in children, except that in adults the clearances tend to be rather higher, with responsiveness. One would be rather worried if a child had a clearance higher than 12.5% IgG, whereas in an adult one would be prepared to try steroids when the IgG clearance is up to 20%. They have the same effect, but slightly shifted upwards.

Mr KENNY: Would the speakers care to comment on methods for the measurement of total protein in urine and CSF?

Dr THOMPSON: There are various methods for the determination of total protein. One commonly sees the sulphosalicyclic acid method used. The problem. with this is that there is a disproportionate ratio between albumin and globulin, and if one is interested in IgG, one does not want to start off on the wrong foot with SSA. One can partially correct for this by adding sodium sulphate to the SSA.

An additional commonly used method is the so-called Lowry method, the Folin copper reagent. The problem with this is that again it measures a number of phenolic derivatives, such as aspirin, thorazine, and various other things that patients with neurological diseases tend to have prescribed in any case. It also measures various peptides.

The bedrock which we use is TCA precipitate followed by a biuret. We have also used the TCA precipitate and Ponceau dye binding which gives slightly lower values, but which in fact is equally satisfactory. However we use poly-ethylene glycol, which is polymerized antifreeze, and what we effectively do is to take 0.2 ml spinal fluid, 2 ml PEG, put it into a boiling water bath for 2 minutes and read it in a nephelometer.

Professor HARDWICKE: I do not think that there is any trouble with urine protein. One must get rid of peptides, and as long as the protein is precipi-tated first – we always use trichloracetic but it is not essential, and we always do a biuret afterwards, because biuret linkages are constant weight related in proteins.

Mr J. G. TEMPLETON (Glasgow): Is anything known about the IgG sub-classes of CSF?

Dr THOMPSON: Yes. A number of people have looked at this. It is principally IgG_1 that is found in the oligoclonal pattern. There are various problems with it. IgG_1 is most antigenic, and the question arises as to whether one should look at the in-effect titration of the different sub-classes.

The short answer is that it is one sub-type. It probably is of one sub-type, although that answer is not sufficiently solid yet.

Index

Acute phase proteins, 157, 239
α_1-antitrypsin, 185, 190, 241
  complement, 162
  haptoglobin, 197–215
  orosomucoid, 197–215
Adjuvant, 39
Affinity (*see* Antisera)
Agar, 4, 5, 8, 9, 10
Agarose, 4, 5, 8, 9, 10, 11
Albumin, 6, 31, 63, 79, 136–148
  analysis, 142–7
    choice of methods, 145
    comparison of methods, 143, 144
    problems, 142
  clinical value, 136
    liver disease, 137
    malnutrition, 136
    protein losing states, 136
  cerebrospinal fluid, 230–4
  normal range, 146
  polymers, 224, 239
  quality control, 147
  standards, 137, 141
    choice of, 141
    NCCLS working group, 141
    purity, 138
  urine, 221, 222, 224
Alpha heavy-chain disease (and *see*
  Heavy chain disease), 121
Amyloidosis, 116
Anaemia, 132
α_1-Antichymotrypsin, 184
Antigen, 150
  binding to antibody, 88
  excess, 18, 26–7, 55
Antisera, 35–49
  absorption, 45
  additives, 46
  affinity, 52
  avidity, 41
  evaluation, 40–5
  fractionation, 45
  processing, 45–7
  production, 36–7, 39
  specificity, 52
  titre, 41, 52

α_1-Antithrombin, 184
α_1-Antitrypsin, 11, 70, 183–193, 232,
  241
  anthropogenetics, 187
  disease, levels in, 190
    emphysema, 190, 191
    fibrosing alveolitis, 190, 192
    glomerulonephritis, 185
    liver cirrhosis, 190–2
    polyarteritis nodosa, 190
    rheumatoid arthritis, 190, 192
  drug therapy, influence of, 190
  electrophoresis,
    crossed immunoelectrophoresis, 185
    isoelectric focussing, 185
    starch gel, 5, 185
  fertility, 193
  inheritance, 188
  oestrogen, effect of, 190, 192, 241
  synthesis, 189
Automated immunoprecipitation, 24–8

Bacteraemia, Gram-negative (*see* Immune
  complex diseases)
Bence Jones protein, 120, 121, 177, 222,
  232
  free light chains, 121, 232
  immunoelectrophoresis, 9
  immunofixation, 12
  investigation of, 123
  myeloma, 117, 123, 124
B-lymphocyte, 88
Breast tumours, 209
Bromocresol green, 79, 145

Carbamylation (*see* electrophoresis)
Carcinoembryonic antigen, 198, 201,
  210, 212–3
Cellogel, 11
Cellulose acetate, 4, 5, 9–12
Cerebrospinal fluid, 230–6
  choroid plexus, 230
Complement, 24, 31, 52, 53, 93, 96,
  149–163, 239
  alternative pathway, 151, 154–6, 159,
    161, 162

anaphylatoxin, 150, 153, 154
binding sites, 152
cellular interactions
  basophils, 150
  cell lysis, 150
  chemotaxis, 150, 153, 154
  eosinophils, 150
  immune adherence, 150, 153, 154
  K (killer) cells, 150
  leukocyte mobilization, 154
  mast cells, 150
  membrane lesions, 154
  mononuclear phagocytes, 150
  neutrophils, 150, 154
  platelets, 150
classical pathway, 151
conversion products, 10, 152
genetic deficiencies of, 158
  detection of, 156
  hereditary angioneurotic oedema,
    159
inactivators, 154
  β1H, 155
  C1 esterase inhibitor, 159, 161, 184
lipopolysaccharides, activation by, 155
measurement, 156, 157
  in disease, 157, 158
  nephritic factor, 156
  opsinization, 159
  vascular permeability, 154
C-reactive protein, 121, 204, 207
Cryoglobulinaemia (see Immune complex
  diseases)
Cryoglobulins, 121, 123, 160, 161
Cryoparaproteins, 121

Drug allergy (see Immune complex
  diseases)
Drugs, antibody response to, 37

Electroendosmosis, 4, 9, 21
Electroimmunoassay (see Immunoelectrophoresis Laurell rocket)
Electrophoresis, 3–15, 220
  carbamylation of proteins, 21
  formylation of proteins, 21
  indications for, 5
  patterns in disease, 7
  scanning, 6
  starch gel, 5

support media, 4
visualization of patterns, 6
zones, 4

Ferritin, 38, 127, 132, 133, 221
  pregnancy, levels in, 238
α_1-Fetoprotein
  obstetrics, 165–176
    amniotic fluid, 166, 167
    fetal serum, 166, 169
    genetic counselling, 170. 171
    maternal serum, conditions
      associated with increase of, 169,
      173, 240
    maternal serum, measurement of,
      171, 174
    multiple pregnancy, 174
    neural tube defects, 167, 169, 171
    Threatened abortion, 174
  oncology, 177–182
    germ cell tumours, 180, 181
    hepatoblastoma, 179
    hepatocellular carcinoma, 178
    other conditions associated with
      increase, 180
Fibrinogen, 121
Fluoronephelometer (see Nephelometry)
Free light chains (see Bence Jones protein)

Gammaglobulins (see Immunoglobulins)
Gc-globulin, 11
Genetic polymorphism, 185
Glomerulonephritis (see Immune complex
  diseases)
Glomerulus, 221

Hageman factor, 184
Haemoglobin, 121, 123, 128
Haemoglobinopathies, 5
Hapten, 37
Haptoglobin, 56, 198–214, 239
  breast tumours, 209–4
  haemoglobin complexes, 234
  lung tumours, 198–209
  oligomers, 234–5
Heavy-chain diseases, 116, 121
Hemopexin, 232
Heparin, 27
Hepatitis B (see Immune complex
  diseases)

Hinge region (*see* Immunoglobulin)
Hormones, antibody response to, 37

Ionic strength, 4
Immune complexes, 158
Immune complex diseases, 158, 160–2
  bacteraemia, Gram-negative, 161, 162
  cryoglobulinaemia, 160, 161
  drug allergy, 160
  glomerulonephritis, 160, 161
  hepatitis B, 160
  malarial nephritis, 160
  polyarteritis nodosa, 160
  polymyalgia rheumatica, 161
  rheumatoid arthritis, 160
  rheumatoid vasculitis, 161
  septicaemia, 162
  serum sickness, 160
  shunt nephritis, 160, 161
  subacute bacterial endocarditis, 160,
    161
  systemic lupus erythematosus, 160,
    161
  vasculitis, 160
Immunization, 39, 40
Immunochemical technique
  accuracy, 52–57, 80
  precision, 57, 80
  reference sera, 70
  sensitivity, 52, 58
  specificity, 52
  standard, 52
Immunodiffusion, radial, 17–21, 54,
    57–9, 157, 166
  influence of molecular size, 20
  Mancini technique, 42
  reversed single, 42
  titration technique, 42
Immunoelectrophoresis, 7–15, 120
  classical, 8
  countercurrent, 9
  Grabar and Williams method, 8, 10
  immunofixation, 10, 11, 120, 237
  Afonso technique, 11
  Laurell rocket technique, 17–21, 54,
    57, 60, 157, 166, 233
  two-dimensional electroimmunoassay,
    10, 18
  transfer, 10

Immunofixation (*see*
    Immunoelectrophoresis)
Immunogen, 37–9
Immunoglobulins, 85–97
  allotypes, 56, 100, 101
  cerebrospinal fluid, 233, 242
  classification, 100, 101
  domains, 86
  function, 88–97
  gammaglobulins, 233–5
  heavy chains, 86
  hinge region, 89
  idiotype, 101, 110, 111
  isoallotype, 101, 110
  isotype, 100
  light chains, 86
  measurement, 21, 31
  secretory, 95
  standardization, 70
  structure, 85–8
  urine, 224
  IgA, 79, 95, 96, 233
    antibodies to, 41
    antigens, 105
    anti-IgA antibodies, 106, 107
    deficiency, 108–9
    secretory, 224
    subclasses, 95
  IgD, 38, 94
  IgE, 38, 96, 97
    myelomas, 97
  IgG, 94, 95, 153, 224, 230–232
    antibodies to, 40, 41
    estimation in cerebrospinal fluid,
      233, 234
    isotypic antigens, 102, 103
    subclasses, 40, 94, 105
  IgM, 38, 92, 153, 233
    antigens, 109
    anti-IgM antibodies, 38
    measurement, problems in, 52, 55,
      59
Inter α-trypsin inhibitor, 184
Iron, 127–132
  binding capacity (TIBC), 129
  binding proteins, 127–133
  deficiency, 129, 132
  metabolism, 128, 129
  overload, 130, 132
Isoelectric points, 4, 21

Lange colloidal gold curve, 233
Laser nephelometry (see Nephelometry)
Laurell rocket technique (see
    Immunoelectrophoresis)
Leukaemia
    monocytic, 116
    myeloid, 224
Lichen myxoedematosis, 116
Light chain diseases, 116
Lung tumour
    serum protein changes, 198–209
Lysozyme, 121, 123, 222, 224
Lymphoma, 116

α_2-Macroglobulin, 224
Macroglobulinaemia of Waldenström,
    116, 124
Malarial nephritis (see Immune complex
    diseases)
Mancini technique (see Immunodiffusion,
    radial)
Membrane receptor, 92, 94
β_2-Microglobulin, 222
Monoclonal proteins (see Paraproteins)
MRC Working Party, 36
Myeloma, 5, 95, 116, 123
    cells in, 111
    non-excreting, 123

Nephelometry, 58, 59, 233
    fluoronephelometer, 24, 25
    laser, 23–33, 42, 145
    sample requirements for, 27
Nephrotic syndrome, 7, 241

Orosomucoid
    breast tumours, 209–214
    cerebrospinal fluid, 232
    lung tumours, 198–209
Ouchterlony double diffusion, 18
Oudin linear diffusion, 18

Pandy technique, 233
Paraproteins, 5, 6, 9, 12, 54, 115–126
    antibodies, as, 116
    benign, 124–6
    cancer, in, 117
    estimation of, 119, 237
    idiopathic, 117
    investigation of, 119

monoclonal, 116, 117
multiple, 122
transient, 122, 238
Passive haemagglutination, 101
Pi system, 185–189
Plasma cells, 88, 96
Plasmin, 184
Polyacrylamide gel, 5
    patterns in cerebrospinal fluid, 234
    patterns in urine, 223, 225
Polyarteritis nodosa (see Immune
    complex diseases)
Polyethylene glycol, 11, 24, 56, 233
Polymyalgia rheumatica (see Immune
    complex diseases)
Pre-albumin, 6, 231
Pregnancy
    associated α_2-glycoprotein (PAG),
        210, 212, 219
Protease inhibitors, 184, 239
Protein
    total measurement of, 242
        Lowry method, 242
        sulphosalicylic acid method, 242
Proteinuria, 219–227, 241
    glomerular, 221, 224
    nephrogenic, 221, 224–6
    overflow, 221, 222–4
    selectivity studies, 241
    tubular, 221, 222
Purpura-hypergammaglobulinaemia, 124
Pyelonephritis, 222

Quality control, 63, 75–80
    national schemes, 78

Radial immunodiffusion technique (see
    Immunodiffusion, radial)
Rhesus antigens, 93
Rheumatoid arthritis (see Immune
    complex diseases)
Rheumatoid vasculitis (see Immune
    complex diseases)

Saliva, proteins in, 96
Salt fractionation, 79, 144
Selectivity studies (see Proteinuria)
Septicaemia (see Immune complex
    diseases)
Serine proteases, 184, 185

Serum sickness (*see* Immune complex diseases)
Shunt nephritis (*see* Immune complex diseases)
Sialic acid, in cerebrospinal fluid proteins, 232
Stains for proteins, 11
Standardization, 63–71, 237
  reference methods, 71
  routine methods, 71
Starch gel (*see* Electrophoresis)
Subacute bacterial endocarditis (*see Immune complex diseases)*
Systemic lupus erythematosus (see Immune complex diseases)

Tamm-Horsfall glycoprotein, 224

Tau protein, 232
Thrombin, 184
Titre (*see* Antisera)
Transferrin, 121, 123, 127, 129–31, 224, 232
Transfusion reactions, 104, 107–8, 238
Turbidimetry, 24

Urinary proteins, 219–26

Vasculitis (*see* Immune complex diseases)

Waldenströms macroglobinaemia (*see* Macroglobinaemia)

Zoning, 121
Zwitterions, 4